ARE YOU READY TO PUT ALL THAT CANCER STUFF BEHIND YOU?

ARE YOU READY TO PUT ALL THAT CANCER STUFF BEHIND YOU?

Using Art Therapy and Affirmations to Heal and Move Forward

Julie Knose

Are You Ready to Put All that Cancer Stuff Behind You? © copyright 2016 by Julie Knose. All rights reserved. No part of this book may be reproduced in any form whatsoever, by photography or xerography or by any other means, by broadcast or transmission, by translation into any kind of language, nor by recording electronically or otherwise, without permission in writing from the author, except by a reviewer, who may quote brief passages in critical articles or reviews.

ISBN-13: 978-1530162604
ISBN-10: 1530162602

Printed in the United States of America
First Printing: 2016
20 19 18 17 16   5 4 3 2 1

Edited by Paper Raven Books
Cover and interior design by Ryan Scheife, Mayfly Design

Contact the author: julieknose@gmail.com
To order, visit Amazon.com

Contents

Introduction . . . . *vii*

PART I: MY CANCER JOURNEY

Chapter One: And So It Begins 3
Chapter Two: Into the Battle 8
Chapter Three: Back to Normal? 15
Chapter Four: No Peace of Mind 22
Chapter Five: Only God Can Judge Me 27
Chapter Six: Walking the Labyrinth 32

PART II: LESSONS I'VE LEARNED

Chapter One: Slow Down 37
Chapter Two: Speak Up 40
Chapter Three: Choose Health 44
Chapter Four: Compassion 46
Chapter Five: Self-Acceptance 49
Chapter Six: Ending Well 53

PART III: ART THERAPY AND WRITING EXERCISES

Introduction 59
Scribble Drawing 60
Emotions Color Wheel 61
Pivotal Moments 62
Dear Cancer Letter 63
Strength Box 64
Flower Mandala 65
Stepping Stones 66

Vision Board 67

Gratitude Jar 68

Gratitude Journal 69

Gratitude Treasure Hunt 70

PART IV: AFFIRMATIONS

Introduction 73

For Healing 77

For Self-Esteem 81

For Courage 85

For Faith 89

PART V: POETRY

Introduction 95

Poems 96

PART VI: MY SPIRITUAL JOURNEY

Chapter One: Meeting Sunny 113

Chapter Two: Message of Hope 117

Chapter Three: Letting Love In 123

Chapter Four: Courage to Fly 132

Chapter Five: Following My Dreams 139

Chapter Six: Heart of the Matter 150

Chapter Seven: Magic and Miracles 160

Chapter Eight: Queen of Gratitude 167

Chapter Nine: Moving Forward 177

Chapter Ten: Happy Dancing 186

Chapter Eleven: Class Is Over 194

Epilogue 199

Afterword 201

Introduction

Before I could put "all that cancer stuff" behind me, I had to put on my big girl panties and deal with it. Treatment sucked. I felt terrible. Cancer is stupid. Everything is different now. I needed time to process my experience. Society tends to rush us through this phase. We don't want to get stuck in our grief or pretend everything is fine. There's a middle path: a way to acknowledge and release pain, choose forgiveness over resentment, and use cancer as a catalyst for personal growth. When it comes to healing, there are no shortcuts.

I wrote this book to share my story, the lessons I've learned, and give you creative tools for your healing journey. There are eleven art therapy and writing exercises to help you express difficult emotions, face cancer-related fears, develop compassion, practice gratitude, and envision a better future. The benefits of art making and journaling include: stress relief, improved coping skills, greater self-awareness, and restored well-being. Now, that's what I call awesome!

There are eighty affirmations to help you build confidence and make positive changes in your life. My poetry will resonate on your frustrating days. Last but not least, the conversations I had with my spirit guide, Sunny, will warm your heart and make you laugh. We cover many topics including: hope, faith, love, courage, dreams, and happiness. I also describe the process of automatic writing, which is how our conversations began. Spirit guides are ethereal beings who offer guidance and protection.

After treatment ended, what I needed most was a wellness coach with a rehabilitation plan. We're shown how to fight cancer, we aren't shown how to heal and move forward. I was sent on my way without any coping tools to deal with the mental, physical, emotional, and spiritual repercussions of cancer treatment. There was no denying the fact that I had just been through a very traumatic experience. There's a good chance cancer treatment has affected you on many levels, too.

The idea of recovery seems easy: rest, recuperate, eat vegetable soup, read books, watch television, eat ice cream, get some exercise, and attend a support group. But when your mind, body, and spirit are wrecked, it isn't an easy fix. I was exhausted, emotional, and resentful. I couldn't keep up with my old pace and the life I once knew moved on without me. They say things happen for a reason, and it takes perspective to see the blessing in disguise. At the time, I felt like a complete failure, like I couldn't even recover from cancer right.

During my recovery, I started making art again remembering the directives I learned in my art therapy classes four years before. I had the tools after all. The Universe had prepared me. Art making became an important part of my healing process. I also found solace in nature walks, yoga, affirmations, and talking with my spirit guide. As more time passed, I was able to gain perspective, make peace with my new normal, and find the silver lining.

If there are two things I hope you learn from this book, it's to TRUST YOUR INTUITION and YOU ARE GOOD ENOUGH. Trust your intuition when it comes to making decisions. Your intuition is very wise and wants the best for you. Your ego can trick you into acts of false bravado. Speak up when something doesn't feel right and ask questions about the long-term effects of treatment. Sometimes, fighting the good fight means slowing down and getting a second opinion. We are unique individuals; we need unique treatment plans.

You are good enough. Even if you're quiet, scared, lonely, confused, and struggling, you're worthy of love and respect. We get into trouble when we doubt our magnificence: we let people treat us badly, we don't apply for promotions or accept dinner invitations; we self-sabotage and play small. We end up blocking the love and abundance that is trying to reach us. We postpone joy because we're waiting to be perfect and have everything figured out. Life is about being vulnerable, taking chances, making mistakes, and learning from them.

Healthy self-esteem gives us the ability to complete projects, get our needs met, and have strong boundaries. Fear creates indecision, scares us into non-action, and destroys confidence. There's a difference between taking time to gather more information and stalling because we're afraid to take the next step. If your choices make you feel empowered rather than depleted you're on the right path. We examine our "I'll be happy when…" stories to make sure we aren't letting ourselves off the hook.

We begin the healing process with self-acceptance and then look for areas of improvement. We don't settle for less, nor do we convince ourselves misery is happiness. Instead of standing still, we take conscious action in the direction of our dreams. By practicing daily affirmations, we take control of our mental chatter and quiet our inner critic. By eliminating self-defeating behaviors, we make progress towards our goals and find that success is possible. We give ourselves permission to be happy and healthy.

The transformation I wish for you is to become a proud survivor who has made peace with the past. Forgiveness, acceptance, gratitude, all of the good stuff is now stored in your heart where it's easily accessible. I know it isn't easy, and some days it's easier to be mad at the world. We soothe the pain with prayer and friendship. We are energized by our creative passions. We fight back because giving up is not an option.

Two more things: FOLLOW YOUR HEART and SHINE YOUR LIGHT. Follow your heart because nobody else can answer your soul calling. Only you know what is true for you. The further I got away from my path, the louder God had to yell. The whispers became hurricanes. Oftentimes, we're afraid to create the life we want because it's not what we're supposed to do, or what our parents have planned for us. We can wait our whole lives for someone else's approval, or we can give ourselves the stamp of approval every day.

Shine your light, my dear! For many years, I deflected compliments, doubted my talents, and dimmed my light. All that did was make me depressed, filled with regret, and robbed the world of my contributions. God created us to be light bearers. We have so much beauty within us, the spark of creativity, and the ability to create life. Now, why on earth should we cower in shame or feel guilty for existing? Your light is your power and strength. Find people who reflect your light back to you rather than people who need you to turn down the brightness.

My intention is to give a voice to the voiceless: patients who have to be brave when their entire world is falling apart; survivors who are expected to return to normal as soon as possible. That patient and survivor was me. There's a fine line between killing cancer cells and harming quality of life. We need to be closely monitored so the damage doesn't outweigh the benefits. It isn't the doctor's fault; that's the ammunition they're given to work with. It isn't the patient's fault; they're following the game plan. The problem is larger than all of us combined. It's a symptom of a much deeper issue: we choose fear over love, and war over peace.

It's hard to write about cancer without sounding incredibly depressing or nauseatingly cheerful. I've tried to balance the heaviness with lightness, because playfulness puts our bodies in a state of relaxation, which activates cellular healing. We think telling the truth will cause us shame, and perhaps it does, but only briefly. In the long run, the truth is the only thing that'll set us free. There's a sickness that lingers long after the illness has been treated. This is the real tragedy; our best treatment leaves many of us disgruntled and debilitated.

Even though we take responsibility for our choices and appreciate the beauty around us, we still have to deal with chronic side effects and the possibility of recurrence. We are brave warriors; the pink ribbon is a tiny consolation. Like kintsugi, the Japanese art of repairing broken pottery with seams of gold, my crescent moon-shaped scar is a beautiful reminder of a difficult time. This is the alchemy of healing: turning struggle into salvation, pain into promise, and folly into faith.

In Part III, Art Therapy and Writing Exercises, you'll need some arts and crafts materials. Suggested supply list: pen, notebook, journal, drawing paper, markers, colored pencils, crayons, scissors, double sided tape, and magazines. For the Strength Box, use a shoebox-sized paper mache box. For the Gratitude Jar, use a large, glass mason jar. You can also buy acrylic paint, brushes, watercolors, and watercolor paper. Choose materials you feel comfortable using. The purpose of art therapy is to express yourself, gain insight, and have fun!

PART I

MY CANCER JOURNEY

CHAPTER ONE

And So It Begins

I was eating the standard American diet. I had repressed anger and resentment towards my alcoholic father. I suffered from depression and low self-esteem. I ended a long-term, loving relationship, losing the person who made everything okay. I moved into a hole-in-the-wall apartment, chased emotionally unavailable men, and smoked a pack of cigarettes a day. I had a stressful job at a drug and alcohol treatment center 1,500 miles from home. My life was going in the wrong direction, and I didn't want to admit it.

The Universe intervened with two terrible storms to teach me valuable lessons. My father's lung cancer diagnosis halted my self-destructive path and brought me back home. My breast cancer diagnosis, two and a half years later, forced me to deal with my emotional baggage and unhealed wounds.

I'm often asked how I found the lump. Accidentally. I stumbled across the lump in November of 2008. It was definitely not a good Christmas present. What in the hell is that? How long have you been there? Just call me Ms. Oblivious.

I wonder if most patients will tell you they knew something was wrong, but couldn't quite put their finger on it. As if the cancer had been working on them, causing symptoms; therefore, finding the lump made complete sense. I knew it was bad news. I got a sinking feeling in the pit of my stomach, the kind you get when you don't make the team or your crush shows up at your party with his new girlfriend. This trumped them.

The lump felt like a marble underneath my skin; it was too hard and distinct to be normal breast lumpiness. I don't have much body fat, so you could see the lump protruding from my skin. The lump was a good inch away from my nipple, near the middle of my chest, not near my armpit. My first thoughts were: I'm going to die. This damn thing is going to kill me. I'm going to need treatment. What in the hell am I going to do now? Just a minute ago everything was fine. Maybe I can rub it away. Go away, please! What did I do wrong? I've messed up this time. I can't weasel my way out of this.

I told my mom, Mary Ann, about the lump. We decided I should go to the gynecologist, who told me the lump was probably nothing, caused by drinking caffeine. She didn't want me to worry. Well, somebody needed to be worried. She thought I was too young to get breast cancer. While most women are over 50, women in their 20s are diagnosed. I was 31 years old. She ordered an ultrasound test which came back negative, a benign finding of fibroadenoma.

So, we let it go. I've since heard a more accurate diagnostic procedure would've been a needle biopsy. I waited six more months. By now it was May of 2009, and the lump wasn't going away. I went to a general surgeon to have the lump removed because it was bothering me. He took one look and without a moment of hesitation said, "Yes, let's get that removed."

Does breast cancer run in my family? Not really. There's a little bit of cancer on both sides of my family. My fraternal grandma, Mary, had colon cancer. My dad, Dave, had lung cancer. Two of my maternal great aunts had breast cancer in their 70s. I wasn't thinking about cancer. I was thinking about getting to work on time, making a haircut appointment, and buying concert tickets. What's for dinner? What's on television? What's the weather going to be like tomorrow? The normal, everyday stuff we take for granted when things are going good. Breast cancer wasn't on my radar.

Friday is not a good day for bad news. Friday has an exciting vibe, because it kicks off the weekend. It's TGIF for a reason; no one ever says "TGIM!" Monday would've been a more appropriate day for bad news; everybody is a grumpy pants already.

I was at my follow-up appointment for the "it's probably nothing" lump the surgeon removed the week before. I don't like needles, blood, or hospitals. I didn't know how to take my pulse or blood pressure. I had no idea what my body did on a daily basis; it seemed to be running fine, and I never bothered to check otherwise. My boss was expecting me in the office after the appointment, so there wasn't time to stop and smell the roses. There wasn't even a Starbucks on my route.

The only consolation, my surgeon was a cutie pie so I didn't mind chatting with him about the weather. Unfortunately, our lighthearted banter ended abruptly. I squirmed in my chair when his cheerful demeanor turned serious. Could the lump be cancer? I took a deep breath.

In 2003, I moved to Santa Fe, New Mexico for graduate school. Since then, my gynecology visits had become sporadic. I wasn't doing monthly breast self-exams or paying attention to the unusual weight loss and fatigue. I was more concerned with putting together an outfit for work that looked professional and caused my co-worker crush, Steve, to do a double take. I also tried to finish the never-ending pile of work on my desk thinking it was imperative to do so.

"You have breast cancer."

"You've got to be kidding me. You're joking, right?" This happens to older women with big breasts. I'm only 31 and wear a 34A bra. I'm a tomboy. I don't like pink. I have my whole life ahead of me. I don't have time for cancer.

I wanted to put the words back into his mouth, turn back time, and start the day over. I could skip the appointment, keep it a secret, and make everything okay again. I should've reminded him it was Friday, and all bets were off. He no longer looked cute to me.

"No, I'm afraid not. This is serious. And you'll need a mastectomy."

"I don't think so." There was no way in hell they were getting chopped off. I've never wanted fake boobs. My breasts are mine; they are small and perfect. Well, they used to be.

The surgeon handed me the pathology report as if I needed proof my life was over. I imagined an F+ written with red marker at the top of the paper. I had failed at the simplest task we're given: to live a healthy life.

"My dad just died of lung cancer. This can't be happening."

"I'm sorry. I wish your mom were here. I assumed she would be."

"She's in Seattle. We didn't think anything was wrong." Just the previous September I had gone with my mom and brother to Yellowstone National Park in Wyoming. We had a great time hiking, exploring the geysers, and taking pictures of the wildlife. We even saw a baby bear cub. I was happy and carefree. I couldn't reconcile that image with where I was now.

"When I removed the lump, it didn't just pop out. I took extra margins for the pathologist. I found out on Wednesday for sure."

"I came here thinking you were going to check the incision, make sure it's healing. I never dreamed you would tell me I have cancer." I started crying.

"I'm sorry. I'll give you the names of two oncologists who have practices nearby."

"Thanks." He did call me the night of the surgery to see how I was doing and remind me to take the Vicodin, but he didn't tell me of his suspicion. Now I know why the recovery was so painful; he took a lot of breast tissue.

I tried to leave the office appearing strong and unaffected. I puffed up my chest like men do when they're trying to be brave. *No big deal; it's just cancer. Oh my God, this is the worst thing in the world. Keep breathing. Put it out of your mind. Hold it together until you get past the ladies at the front desk. Breathe.*

Nope. I broke down sobbing, louder than a fire truck siren, shoulders heaving, looking through my purse for a tissue. I was ushered to a private room to compose myself before I could drive home.

"Are you going to be okay?" the nurse asked. I told her yes even though I knew it'd be a long time before I was okay again. I went to the ladies' restroom to cry in peace. I must've gone into shock because, when I looked in the mirror, I was white as a ghost and the tears had disappeared. My mind was protecting me until all of the information could be digested.

I walked outside to locate my car. It was a warm, sunny day, but everything looked different now. People walked by me. Their world was the same; my world had changed. Like children tumbling down a hill, my thoughts increased their speed. *Something bad just happened. The lump was cancer. I'm going into work; they can help me. I have to tell someone. I can't be alone right now. Everything's going to be okay. This wasn't the vacation I was hoping for; this wasn't the future I had in mind. Turn on the radio and find a happy song.*

I drove to work, found a parking space, walked inside the building, and handed my boss, Carolyn, the pathology report. We talked about breast cancer, how serious it was, and getting time off for treatment. I called the female oncologist the surgeon referred me to and set up an appointment for the following week. I was glad to see her oncology practice was a short drive from my mom's house.

My co-worker, Terri, and I took a break like we always did. This time we talked about how nothing would ever be the same again. She sat with me while I called my mom who cut her vacation short and flew home the next day.

I didn't work much that afternoon; I made some photocopies, went home, and cried. The next few weeks were filled with doctor appointments, treatment planning, and breaking the news to family and friends.

CHAPTER TWO

Into the Battle

Highlights from my pathology report dated 06/02/2009: Breast mass, right-excision with margins, invasive ductal carcinoma, grade 3 extending to surgical margins. (Grade 3 is a high grade, unfavorable. The cells are poorly differentiated.) Lymphatic invasion is identified. The tumor is estrogen receptor positive, greatest dimension 2.1 cm.

After the genetic counseling and risk assessment, I tested negative for the BRCA gene mutation. After the sentinel node biopsy, I learned 1/11 lymph nodes tested positive for cancer cells.

Cancer staging is based on several factors: tumor size, lymph node involvement, and whether or not it has spread. Stage 0 is DCIS, ductal carcinoma in situ, meaning the cancer is not invasive and will not spread. Stage IV is advanced breast cancer, which is also called metastatic because it has spread to other organs in the body.

I was diagnosed with stage II breast cancer on Friday, June 5th 2009. Stage II is considered an early stage that responds well to treatment. I had several different scans and tests to make sure the cancer hadn't spread elsewhere. I closed my eyes every time a needle came near me. The nurses probably thought I was funny.

I was naïve, scared, and ready to fight. I thought I would bounce back like nothing happened. I underestimated how aggressive modern medical treatment would be and the effect it would have on my body, mind, and spirit.

I went to the plastic surgeon information appointment. The sight of the implants made me sick to my stomach. When I started bawling my eyes out, I think she got the message that I wasn't going to be her next patient. I'm not sure why I was able to get pumped full of poison while the thought of losing my breasts was unbearable. My breast cancer surgeon,

Dr. H., was able to get clear margins after the lumpectomy, so I didn't need the mastectomy after all.

My cancer treatment consisted of three surgeries: lumpectomy, two re-excisions to get clear margins, and a sentinel node biopsy/port installation. I completed four months of chemotherapy and six weeks of radiation. I had many side effects: anemia, peripheral neuropathy, bone pain, blurred vision, fibromyalgia, cognitive dysfunction, fatigue, nausea, pulsatile tinnitus, and lymphedema. Some have gotten better, but some are chronic.

I didn't take Tamoxifen, although it was recommended as hormone therapy because my tumor was estrogen receptor positive. Tamoxifen is a pill taken for five years to reduce the amount of estrogen in the body. Sometimes, I regret not taking it and wonder if I made a mistake. I refused the easiest part of treatment, but at the time I was dealing with so many side effects that I couldn't handle the idea of having any more.

While I'd like to paint a rosy picture of chemotherapy, I won't. For one, it'd be a lie, and two, it'd be disrespectful to cancer survivors who've endured the experience. I don't want to discourage patients from getting treatment, but I have to give my honest opinion. Chemotherapy is barbaric and inhumane; a somewhat tolerable torture that causes heart and nerve damage. Is that the price we have to pay? I don't know.

It's hard to be grateful for something that caused me pain and misery. I was brave enough to sit in the chair and face the unknown. I remember a short conversation I had with the male oncology nurse, David, as he walked me back to the treatment room.

"You know you don't have to smile," he said in a low, serious tone. I think he was trying to tell me I didn't have to be so brave.

"I'm smiling so I don't cry." The words tumbled out of my mouth, surprising us both. I wondered what he'd think of me when my hair fell out.

I felt a strong, silent bond with the other patients, because we were in the same boat. Our treatment plans might've been different, but we were battling the same scary disease. We were going through something that would change us forever.

I began to experience irregular periods, mood swings, food cravings, irritability, and frequent crying that felt like a never-ending case of PMS.

My body tried to go into early menopause, but my periods have resumed. I was a nightmare to live with; it felt like there was an angry beast inside of me who wanted to break things and destroy the house. This could've been caused by the steroids they were giving me to keep my energy levels up. My mom put up with way more than she should have.

I wanted to throw up after chemo, but I wasn't able to because of the pre-meds, specifically an anti-nausea medication called Emend, a powerful little pill that tells your mind, "No, you don't have a toxic chemical cocktail in your bloodstream. You're just fine." I only threw up once on a Sunday evening after my Thursday treatment. I hate vomiting, and I'm terrible at it, so I'm lucky it wasn't a common occurrence.

Chemotherapy is a yucky feeling, like waiting for the war to be over. I told myself, "I can handle this. I can tolerate this. No big deal. This is for the best. This is what people do. I've got to keep going no matter what. I have to be brave."

I received four doses of Adriamycin appropriately nicknamed The Red Devil because it's red in color, and I was shaking hands with death after one dose. Don't underestimate Adriamycin. Four doses is the maximum amount you can get, because it's so toxic. After the second dose, my hair fell out in clumps. It was a very unsettling experience, because my hair was no longer attached to my scalp. I put on my baseball cap to keep it from falling out, which obviously didn't work. Instead of having clumps of hair everywhere, my mom helped me shave my head. Bald is beautiful!

I wanted to stop after the third dose, but I soldiered ahead. I didn't want the last dose. I knew it was strangling my heart. I remember the night I thought I was going to die. My mom and I were watching the cooking show, *Chopped*. I started feeling horrible and couldn't watch the rest of the show. I went upstairs to get ready for bed. When my mom came to check on me, I told her, "Maybe we should go to the emergency room." It felt like my head was going to explode, and I started seeing white light. I grabbed my head and prayed for relief. At that point, I must've passed out. When I woke up the next morning, I felt better.

The next chemo drug I received was Taxol; it was a clear liquid. I found Taxol easier to tolerate than Adriamycin. Taxol felt like the flu whereas Adriamycin felt like I was on my deathbed. You can get more doses of Taxol and take it weekly, but it causes peripheral neuropathy. I thought the numb, burning sensation in my hands and feet was a temporary side effect that would go away after treatment ended. When I finally told my oncologist about it, after the ninth dose, she declared me done with treatment.

We have a lot of different nerves: motor, sensory, and autonomic. Unfortunately, all of these are affected by Taxol. The pins and needles sensation made walking on cement painful. It can take several years for your nerves to heal and regenerate. It's been five years and although it's better, I still have neuropathy.

After treatment ended, it felt like the inside of my body had been beaten with a metal baseball bat. I'd lie on the couch aching all over; it was a pain I couldn't ignore or alleviate. Chemotherapy also wreaked havoc on my circulation. My blood pressure was low and my pulse was high. Lymph fluid accumulated in my legs, blood pooled in my feet, and it drove me crazy. My body was having trouble functioning.

I did this to myself. I let them do this to me. If this is living, I'd rather be dead. The fact that I couldn't undo the damage was the hardest part. My once beautiful body, which I didn't think twice about, betrayed me and became my prison. When I looked in the mirror, instead of seeing a vibrant young woman, I saw Beetlejuices's twin sister (if he had one) complete with ghostly paleness, green mold, and dark under-eye circles.

~

Compared to chemotherapy, radiation was a breeze. I had to lie down on a table five days a week while a machine came on, made funny noises, and zapped me with a laser beam. I'm sure it had more complicated names and terms for what actually happened, but for once I just didn't want to know. My cheerful optimism was gone, replaced with apathy and disgust for my new reality.

The radiation lab wasn't a busy place. The sterile hallways had a cold, lonely feeling. I guess getting radiation is not on the top of anyone's to-do list. I barely remember the short-term side effects. They weren't very bothersome: a sunburn and peeling. But radiation is like overeating; it's a cumulative effect that takes awhile to notice. And once again, I thought I'd walk away unscathed, like I had some special bulletproof vest.

Radiation caused a feeling of exhaustion incomparable to anything I'd experienced before. It's difficult to explain, even harder to fathom, and a nightmare to live. You don't slow down on purpose; you are slowed down. My body had become a toxic waste dump, and the fog was very heavy indeed. I worried the fatigue was going to consume me. Even brushing my teeth was a chore my body could barely tolerate.

I needed to get some rest, but not too much. A nap turned into a pile of bricks lying on top of me, and it took all of my strength to get up from the couch. It felt like the treatment had aged me forty years. I was in my own private hell, because I didn't know if the fatigue would lessen. I hoped and prayed that it would.

I'm not a lazy person. I've never been a couch potato. I'm one of those people who can't sit still for very long because I have too much nervous energy. Everything took so much longer. I felt like I was in slow motion. I had to give myself a twenty-minute head start to pull myself up the stairs, go to the bathroom, and get back downstairs to watch *Jeopardy*. Before cancer, this would've taken five minutes. Supposedly, slow and steady wins the race. Having the speed of the tortoise when you're used to being the hare is a lesson in faith and patience.

The best way to counteract fatigue is to start an exercise program. I've always loved to exercise, so it wasn't a chore in that sense. I went for a walk one day by myself. Not even half-way through the neighborhood, my body was done. I was actually done before I left the house, but I was hoping to kick it into high gear like the good old days. I worried I wouldn't have the energy to make it home, and I'd be stuck there forever, or until my mom realized I hadn't returned home. I didn't have my cell phone with me, so I stood in the shade hoping my energy would return. After several minutes of deliberation, I decided to resume walking; it felt like I was pulling an elephant behind me. Those three short blocks to get back home were a marathon.

When the radiologist said I was going to feel tired for about a year, he wasn't joking. Tired didn't even begin to describe it. Simple things made me smile, like being at the grocery store picking out bananas and tomatoes. It took all of my strength to get dressed and leave the house. I looked like a real hot mess and never would've gone to the grocery store like that before cancer. Imperfections paled in comparison to the task at hand. Although I still cared what people thought, and felt frustrated with my vanity. When I accidentally dropped a cucumber on the floor because I was nervous, I was grateful for the lady standing next to me who said, "That's the one that got away." A huge smile lit up my face, and I replied, "There have been a few that got away." I didn't feel good, and that trip to the grocery store was a big deal for me; it was a victory!

Journal Entries:

October 18, 2009

Today is Sunday, I got my first dose of Taxol on Thursday; it's not as bad as Adriamycin. I'm having cold chills. I don't have a big appetite. I'm losing weight and muscle. I'm going to have to work out hard core. Doctor said neuropathy is possible, numbness in hands and feet.

All of my teeth hurt. My hearing is muffled, which is really annoying. I don't know how loud or quiet I'm talking. Blood pressure was 90/60. Treatment was halted for a week because my counts were too low. Watch for constipation. Dr. W. told me I'm anemic, chemo depleted my red blood cells. I'm going to eat more spinach.

Look for a cancer support group. FROG = Fully Rely On God. Giving up hope is never the answer. Return to work. Stay motivated. Set goals. Get out of my sweatpants. My heart seems fragile now. Fatigue and bone pain are awful. Push past them.

I need some normalcy, times when I'm not the patient who is sick with cancer. I need to be seen as competent, not always taken care of, babied, and asked how I am doing. The patient and the caregiver need time apart; separation is good. When I get better, I can move out and get on with my life.

November 5, 2009

Mom said that I did well today. We went out for breakfast after treatment; I got blueberry pancakes, my favorite. I'm too nervous to eat beforehand and then I don't feel like eating afterward once the chemo starts working its magic. Last week, I cried during treatment, the reality of the situation finally caught up with me. The nurses let me cry, they didn't rush over to fix my sadness. You can't be brave every minute of the day. And sometimes, crying is the bravest thing we can do.

JANUARY 18, 2010

The other oncologist told me it'll take six-to-nine months to feel back to normal. I don't think I'll ever feel back to normal, maybe years from now. He's one of those optimistic doctors. I finished chemo on New Year's Eve. What a weird way to end the year. I feel exhausted and emotional. I'm starting radiation soon. I have to keep fighting even though I want to give up. I need motivation. Some people have it much worse, I should be thankful. I'm scared that I won't recover from this nightmare. My hair is growing back slowly. I like short hair. Someday, I'll have a ponytail again. No one understands. Don't tell them I've gone crazy. I'm having a hard time and that's okay.

CHAPTER THREE

Back to Normal?

I finished radiation treatment on March 5th 2010. I returned to work two months later. It was time to come back, they said, or my position would be given away. How was I feeling? Like death rolled over and stomped on me. I couldn't believe how bad I felt. I didn't want to lose my job. I needed to prove to the world that I had survived the war. Unfortunately, the treatment took more than I had to give. Chemotherapy side effects are immediate, radiation fatigue hits hard after treatment ends. For me, the combination of the two was more than my body could handle.

I wanted to put "all that cancer stuff" behind me. I liked my job and co-workers. The routine was good for me. I didn't want it to be true that the treatment had caused something bad to happen. I didn't want there to be anything wrong. I wanted to go back to the way things were when I was invisible in the insurance company cubicle sorting mail and answering phones. For gosh sakes, they need me, I'm good at what I do.

I had already gone through hell, so my tolerance for pain and abnormal sensations was pretty high. Treatment was over; why did I still feel bad? I hoped the pain would go away if I just kept going and tried to forget about it. No such luck.

Finally, I told my mom what was happening. We ended up calling them "the headaches" because we needed a name for them, but they were much worse than any headache I'd ever had, and they were at the base of my skull/top of my neck, not on my forehead. It felt like there were knives slashing back and forth. It felt like gravity was pushing me down.

The only time the pain went away was when I would lay down. My body was having trouble functioning in the upright position. Sitting or standing for an extended period of time proved difficult. Nevertheless, I continued to work and tried to go out with my friends, even though the pain was nearly incapacitating. I remember my friend, Christen, could tell I wasn't feeling good, and she commented that my eyes looked glassy. As if I weren't dealing with enough pressure to recover quickly, now I had this weird pressure literally bringing me down.

After two months of trying to hang in there, I had to face reality—the pain wasn't going away, and I couldn't do my job anymore. I had to stop and admit there was a serious problem. This hurt my pride, and I felt like a complete failure. I took the blame for something that wasn't my fault.

My body needed to rest; otherwise, the pain would never go away. I'd get my shower and then lie down. I'd eat and then lie down. I'd stand at the sink trying to brush my teeth before the pain became incapacitating. If I had an appointment, I'd get ready and then lie down until we had to leave. The headaches were taking over my life. Ironically, I had worked briefly during chemotherapy, wearing my baseball cap, trying to maintain a strong connection with my job. We were more worried about life after treatment rather than how the treatment was affecting me.

While I was getting treatment, two positions in the clerical department were dissolved and mine was one of them. Having been with that department for a year and a half, I knew my job pretty well. I was promoted and transferred to another department with the duties of a claims adjuster. This was exactly what I didn't want, and why I had chosen to be in the clerical department. I had no passion for insurance, didn't understand it, and no part of me wanted to go through training. When I returned from leave, I had to learn a new job in a new department with a new supervisor. Maybe if the transfer had happened before cancer, I would've been able to figure it out. I was getting further away from my creative path. It took the headaches and my unhappiness to force me to quit in July of 2010. Staying at that job wasn't helping me or them.

I went to several sympathetic neurologists. At least they had heard of similar cases, and I didn't feel like I was going crazy. One of them looked at me like, "Well, what did you expect to happen?" And then he told me, "The treatment probably caused it, and there's no magic bullet to fix it." They finally agreed that it resembled a spinal tap or epidural headache. "You could be leaking spinal fluid." I didn't even know I had spinal fluid. By this point, I was going out of my mind because I had to be upright during these doctor visits. They suggested doing a complicated procedure: a CT myelogram, lumbar puncture, and injecting a radioactive tracer to locate the leak. I don't like surgery and that sounded dreadful.

They offered me a blood patch which I refused. I was at my breaking point. I didn't know what to do. I couldn't risk one more complication; the pain was already unbearable. I needed a remedy, yet their option didn't sound like a good one. I had about all I could take of doctors and their treatments. I think they could sense my frustration.

The neurologist's advice was to lie down for three days, only getting up to eat meals, and see if it got better. He also suggested using a very flat pillow when I slept. I continued to lie down as much as possible, because it gave me relief, and I was hoping to heal whatever was wrong. The next thing I knew, I had become bed-ridden. My body was getting more used to being horizontal than vertical.

I was a soccer player and this period of inactivity was difficult for me. I had a lot of time on my hands to think about things. One day, I brought my markers and sketchbook to bed with me. It dawned on me that I could use what I'd learned in my art therapy classes on myself. As if the Universe was telling me, "You're suffering, and you have the tools to express yourself. Do you think we'd take you through the storm unprepared?" I made a scribble drawing, which turned into a flower mandala. It was an awesome feeling to be making art again, but the flowers looked sad and pitiful. I made more flowers and butterflies, each one showing my struggle quite clearly. I tried to make them happy, I wanted them to be happy, but they weren't because I wasn't. I hung them on my bedroom wall as if to say, "This is how I'm feeling. The pain is outside of me; I've released it. I'm going to be okay. It might not be today, but someday."

When I went to see my oncologist, she warned me that if I stayed in bed any longer, I'd become an invalid. This scared me. I began staying up a little more each day, two to four hours at a time before the pain forced me to lie down again. Next, I split the day in two, lying down for a nap from four to six pm. We were erring on the side of caution, easing back into being upright all day. I needed to push myself and build my stamina. I thought to myself, "It has to get better, because it can't get any worse."

Transitioning slowly made the most sense. I was still exhausted from the radiation treatment, so it wasn't difficult to take a nap. During this time, I read books and wrote the fiction story. My body was finally getting the rest it needed, but I had a long way to go before I reached my highest level of function. I needed to strengthen my heart.

My mom and I started walking at Forest Fair Mall, once a popular, thriving shopping center when I was in high school, now nearly vacant except for a few stores. The mall had a sad, cold, empty feeling. Even the dust bunnies, which accumulated in the corners, felt neglected and abandoned. As we walked down the dimly lit corridors, I could hear echoes of good times and laughter; it felt like my life. I had gotten so far out of shape that we had to walk slowly, and the senior citizen mall walkers lapped us; it was a humbling experience. We walked for 30 to 45 minutes several days a week, and I began to feel much better. When the weather turned warmer, we walked outside at the cemetery where my dad is buried.

I haven't talked too much about my dad, but his death was my first wake-up call. Back in December of 2006, I was living in Santa Fe, New Mexico, my dad called to tell me he'd been diagnosed with stage IV lung cancer. He'd been smoking and drinking for many years, so this didn't surprise anyone. Nevertheless, it broke my heart. I packed my bags as soon as we hung up the phone. There wasn't a question in my mind about where I needed to be. My brother was living in Park City, Utah, and we both flew home the first week of January.

That was a wise move. My dad's oncologist told my mom to have the kids come home. My dad was in the hospital. He'd gotten one round of chemotherapy which wreaked havoc on his already compromised health. His legs were thick with edema. He had a doctor for every organ in his body. When I walked into his room, my knees nearly buckled and tears filled my eyes. They were trying to save him; if only he'd saved himself a long time ago. I was so mad at him. Why didn't he want to live?

He wanted to live.

After a few months, they moved him to hospice for palliative care, which means no more treatment, giving him some quality of life in the remaining time. One night in his morphine-induced state he said, "You're going to stand there and watch me walk away."

The day he died he made a face that said, "I'm done." He had a moment of clarity. I saw him fight to stay with us. He was tired of being in pain. He made peace with God. He asked for forgiveness. He was scared;

I saw it in his eyes. He died four months after I got his call. I moved back home to Ohio for good to be near my mom. There was nothing left for me in Santa Fe.

It takes time to wrap our hearts around the truth. In the beginning, it was easier to pretend my dad wasn't dead. He's away on a business trip. Nope. My dad's in heaven. He's allowed to visit occasionally when one of us needs encouragement. Every once in awhile, I'll look out the window and see someone who looks almost exactly like him walking on the bike path. I silently scream out, "Dad!" as the tears stream down my face. I don't know if he likes the person I've become. Some days, I don't like her either.

While we continued to walk near my dad's grave, I decreased my nap time to 30 minutes a day, so I could elevate my feet and relieve the edema in my legs. No one but my mom understood the struggle I was going through to regain my strength. One night, she made bean and rice burritos for dinner because they're my favorite. I was trying to gain weight because I'd lost so much during treatment. I went downstairs and saw the delicious dinner, but I was overcome with sadness. I sat down and started crying. I didn't know if things were ever going to get better. My situation felt hopeless. My mom reassured me that everything was going to be okay. It took awhile but she was right.

My mom's a smart lady.

After six months of letting my body heal naturally, by the grace of God, the pain went away, and I'm very grateful. I'll never know for sure what was wrong: leaking spinal fluid, low pressure headaches, dysautonomia, or orthostatic hypotension. I do know it was treatment induced and, therefore, in a league of its own. Even though I was able to sit in a chair for an extended period of time, I worried the headaches would come back; there was no way I could go through that again. I tried to be constantly moving or lying down because I thought this was the answer.

I didn't realize how important my heart was until it stopped functioning properly. I wondered if I would ever live again without worrying about the basics. I began body monitoring by checking my pulse and blood pressure. I worried about the blood pooling in my feet because I thought my brain wouldn't have enough. It was a lonely time for me. I slowly began to trust my body as more time passed and the pain didn't come back.

The good news, I can sit in a chair now without worrying and even though an afternoon nap would be awesome, I don't take them very often. There are times when I need to rest, but I continue working. I either push myself too hard or not hard enough. I'm trying to listen to my body and find a good balance. I was on a mission to get my physical strength back because that was my way of telling the cancer it didn't win.

Journal Entries:

SEPTEMBER 23, 2010

I've lost my mind. I've lost everything that was important to me. I don't know what the day will hold. I'm a million miles away, I don't have anyone. I'm ugly and grotesque. I fool myself into believing there's a place for me in this world. I fool myself into believing they really care. I don't worry less, I worry more.

I have to find a way out of this mess and make the best of the time I have left. Be as productive as possible. Stay far away from the people who drag me down, like I can get any lower. My life is no longer simple like yours. I think the chemo damaged my whole body. People want to see beauty and confidence. I look like a leper. I feel like a toxic waste dump.

Don't tell me you care. You wouldn't have taken me there to get poisoned. This writing is pointless, no one cares and evil prevails. We promote war instead of peace. We tell each other lies because the truth comes with a price. Please God, give me the strength to carry on, a sign that things will get better. I don't want to be damaged forever.

NOVEMBER 8, 2010

I'm having suicidal thoughts. Do I have a plan? No. Well, a few ideas: car crash or pills. I don't like heights or the idea of hanging. My luck, I'd probably mess it up. I always worry at the last minute I'd regret my decision, but then it'd be too late.

Whenever I think about suicide, I feel like I'm disrespecting God and being ungrateful for my life. God knows I'm struggling. He understands. I'm having trouble sitting and standing. I don't know whether it's the heart or nerve damage. I'm depressed. My quality of life is a joke. I have to act like I'm okay because my mom is tired of hearing about it. Everyone else works after cancer treatment, why can't you?

Do you know how difficult it is to be positive when you're in pain? I need to get some fresh air. I haven't been able to gain weight. The neuropathy is painful. I feel it in my hands and feet. I don't wish this on my worst enemy. I pray my nerves can heal and regenerate.

November 12, 2010

I have to find a reason to live. I'm so damn tired of trying. I'd rather be dead, because I don't want to live like this. My mom is in denial. She's only concerned with me getting out of her way. I'm a burden to her, a pebble in her shoe. I'm comforted by the fact that suicide will give me a way out. The pain has become my friend in a way. I was afraid of it for a long time.

I don't know what's wrong. Am I leaking spinal fluid? I'm scared and alone. I don't trust anyone anymore, especially doctors. Most days, I welcome death, and other days I fool myself into believing I should continue living. They scare you with the cancer diagnosis, make you vulnerable, and unable to think straight. No, I don't want cancer, but the long-term side effects aren't a walk in the park, either. I can complain about how bad I feel until I'm blue in the face. I can record my blood pressure until I run out of paper; it won't make a difference. I have to live with the consequences of my choices.

CHAPTER FOUR

No Peace of Mind

Dealing with physical ailments was bad enough; developing severe anxiety further delayed my recovery. After everything I'd been through, I shouldn't have been afraid of anything, yet I'd become afraid of everything. Instead of returning to a normal level of functionality, my body was stuck in fight-or-flight mode like a scared rabbit scanning the field for danger, muscles clenched, eyes wide with fear. I wanted to protect myself from something bad happening again.

The war was over, but I had a bad case of shell shock and battle fatigue. The armor that usually protected my sensitivities was gone. Traumatic memories are stored in the body and get triggered by everyday things. The problems weren't outside of me; I was creating them from the inside. I knew the things I worried about were silly, yet my fears were real and the consequences felt dire.

Post-traumatic stress disorder (PTSD) is caused by experiencing or witnessing an event that causes serious harm, followed by feelings of helplessness and horror. Symptoms can start within three months of the traumatic event and interfere with living a normal life. I began to experience all three categories: reliving, avoiding, and increased arousal.

I started getting triggered by the antibacterial Softsoap bottle sitting on the bathroom counter. It took me awhile to realize what was happening and why being in the bathroom caused me distress. The Softsoap was a clear liquid in a clear container. The chemotherapy was a clear liquid in a clear bag. They looked similar enough for the memory to get triggered. When I told my doctor about the strange association, she said some survivors can't sit in a recliner anymore because it reminds them of getting treatment.

I decided to control the situation by making sure the Softsoap was sitting in the "right spot." If it got moved from its designated place, I had to move it back. Before leaving the bathroom, I'd double-check to make sure it was standing upright. If anyone made a mess and the soap ended up on the counter, it felt like an oil spill and caused me anxiety. My rational mind knew the soap was harmless, and luckily I was able to wash my hands. It was the sight of the container that bothered me, not the soap.

Interestingly, I wasn't getting triggered by the moisturizing Softsoap in the kitchen because it was an opaque liquid. I begged my mom to stop using the clear kind and switch to the opaque kind, and this helped a lot. Now I realize there are containers that aren't see-through, which are even better because I can't see the liquid at all.

Instead of getting better, I got worse. I started having panic attacks almost every day. They're very serious; not to be taken lightly. Once I started having them, I started fearing them, too. The anxiety is so intense that it feels like you're dying. The panic attacks happened in my bedroom, right before I went into the bathroom to put on my deodorant. It felt like performance anxiety; I was afraid I'd mess up and do it wrong. I couldn't believe such a simple task was causing me so much trouble. My friends were all at work while I had just managed to apply deodorant. My life had slowed down to a standstill, again.

Trauma does strange things to a person; it destroys peace of mind and shuts down our capacity to experience joy. Similar to the way depression causes life to be seen through a distorted lens, trauma creates a foreboding future. I stopped talking because no one could hear me. I trashed my room breaking all the things I loved. I figured I might as well make an even bigger mess because everything is ruined now.

This wasn't healthy. I broke my silence and went to see a therapist. She helped me process my cancer experience and rebuild my confidence. I moved into an apartment in December of 2012. This was a big deal because it meant regaining my independence. My mom and I were able to move from caregiver-patient to a mother-daughter relationship again.

Since moving out of my mom's house, the panic attacks are few and far between. I'm able to apply deodorant without a problem. I take a few deep breaths and follow my sequence. I've had more wins than losses, so this gives me confidence. It's not a big deal anymore. I thank my lucky stars that things are much better now.

My first year in the apartment went okay. I talked to my spirit guide and worked on the manuscript. In the summer, I went swimming in the gorgeous saltwater pool. I took walks to clear my head and stretch my legs. I found a weeping willow tree and small pond where I could reconnect with nature. I took photos of nature and found photography to be another passion of mine. I opened up a Twitter account and made some new friends.

My second year in the apartment didn't go quite as well. I quit seeing my therapist and my issues resurfaced. A common refrain I heard from my mom when we talked about the past and all the things I used to do, "That was back when nothing bothered you."

Obsessive Compulsive Disorder (OCD) can be described like this—a person has unwanted thoughts (obsessions) and then has to perform repetitive behaviors (compulsions) to relieve anxiety. My obsessive thoughts revolved around a fear of contamination and being harmed again. My compulsive behaviors included rinsing my hands, folding clothes, putting in my ponytail holder, checking faucets, and parking my car. I had to follow a certain sequence when showering and getting dressed. It's okay to have a routine and do things a certain way because it's more efficient. It crosses the line into OCD when it becomes time-consuming and prevents you from enjoying life.

I had a ritual to leave the bathroom and apartment, which we referred to as "doing my checks." I repeated weird mantras in my mind like, "Coffee pot, check, stove, check, towel, check. Soap is standing, soap is my friend. Blue door, blue door, blue door, all is well in my world." Although it's important to make sure the coffee pot is turned off and the doors are locked, my checking was excessive. By the time I left the house, I was late and frazzled. When my anxiety is low, the checking goes quickly. When my life feels "out of control" that's when I look around for things to control. This is an important realization for me. When I'm feeling confident, I don't second-guess myself.

In the wintertime, my phobia was stepping on road salt. I wore shoes that didn't have grooves on the bottom, so I couldn't track the salt into my apartment. I had to think of them as magic crystals every time I heard them crunch under my shoes. I was obsessed with the idea of things being either clean or dirty, and in my mind dirty things were harmful and couldn't touch clean things.

My anxiety became debilitating. Trying to protect myself from harm caused me more harm. My quality of life slowly deteriorated. I missed holidays, my brother's wedding in Utah, and the birth of my niece, Emma. I never got another full-time job, which hurt my pride. The longer I stayed isolated, the worse I became. Somebody needed to file a missing person report because I was lost and alone. I felt like I had let everyone down, and I was going to let myself down, too.

My need for control had shrunk my world into something vaguely resembling a life. I wouldn't let anyone into my apartment except for the maintenance man to do repairs. I no longer had fun, because I couldn't let my guard down for that long. The list of things I couldn't do grew longer.

Even a short trip to the grocery store with my mom became a huge ordeal. We couldn't park next to another car. I had to be careful where I walked so that I didn't step in anything. In my mind, the world had become a dangerous place with possible contaminations everywhere. The thought of something touching and harming me again caused me serious distress.

If I drove, I kept re-parking the car until I had either driven myself crazy, drawn attention to myself, or found a suitable space. I watched other people park their car once and go into the store, oblivious to the torment in my mind. I hated driving home from the grocery because it meant I'd have to park the car. I spent the five-minute drive visualizing myself pulling into the space. I had to make sure I was parked equidistance from each line before I could turn off the engine. I did a final check before going into the building. If anyone interrupted the final check, I'd have to do it again.

I stopped driving my car for awhile because the pressure to park perfectly in the space was so intense. I knew the other cars weren't parked perfectly, and mine didn't have to be either, but for some reason it felt like life-or-death. One night, coming home from my mom's house, I kept re-parking the car and had a panic attack. I was embarrassed that I was having so much trouble, because my neighbors could see me from their windows. I wanted to go into my apartment because I was getting tired, and it was getting dark outside making it even harder to see the lines. Somehow, I think out of sheer exhaustion, I made peace with my parking space and went inside. Luckily, it got to the point where I could park perfectly, or near perfectly, the first time. I think the angels started intervening, because I kept praying, "Parking miracle find me now."

After everything I'd been through, to be stuck in my house was downright depressing. The worst part was I understood the psychology behind it and still couldn't find my way out. My worries were exhausting my mom, too. Gone were the days of being flexible and spontaneous; everything had to be preplanned. I knew things were bad when I got excited about seeing a puddle of water on the side of the road.

It's hard being honest about my struggle, because society views struggle as weakness and no one likes to appear weak. Looking back, I can't believe I caused myself so much unnecessary trouble. I had too much time on my hands. I developed maladaptive coping mechanisms to deal with the trauma I had been through. The OCD was a red herring for not living my life, and the behaviors would fade away if my life were busier.

In January of 2015, I got myself back into therapy to deal with these issues. My mom found the therapist and drove me to the appointment. Therapy isn't easy; it's a commitment to taking responsibility and making changes. My therapist, Dr. R., is supportive and encouraging. Sometimes, all it takes is one person who believes in us then we're motivated to get better. Therapists provide a safe environment for healing to occur. Therapists help us to set specific, measurable, and attainable goals.

CHAPTER FIVE

Only God Can Judge Me

I looked out the window and saw a plastic bag stuck in the branches of a small tree. The wind was trying to set the bag free, but it was really stuck. It was a good analogy of depression. We're the bag, the tree represents depression, and the wind is our support system. The longer the bag stays attached to the tree, the more damaged it becomes. The longer we stay depressed, the harder it is to get unstuck. I was rooting for the bag to get unstuck, yet wishing the angry wind would calm down. If we're not ready to change, even our well-intentioned support system can do more harm than good. I've felt like the bag many times: not where I'm supposed to be and struggling to get free.

People have varying degrees of depression; some need medication to function while others do not. What works for me might not work for you. I'm not an expert on mental health; I can only speak from my experience. I've been on anti-depressants, and I wasn't any happier. Sure, my neurons were constantly soaking in serotonin, so I couldn't hit the low notes, but listening to a soundtrack composed entirely of high notes didn't sound right, either.

I couldn't cry at my dad's funeral. It's okay to feel sad and go through periods of sadness. My little, blue Zoloft pill must've peaked during the funeral. I was probably in denial and dissociating, too. When I tried to go back on anti-depressants after treatment ended, they made me extremely dizzy. I can't tolerate them now. I have to find natural remedies for depression: exercise, sunlight, friendship, nutrition, and creative hobbies.

Depression should be seen as a signal that change needs to occur, not that we must cheer up immediately. Heaven forbid we turn off the television long enough to share our feelings or have an intelligent conversation. People who have mental disorders are often very creative;

otherwise, how on earth could we do what we do? We laugh about it, but the stigma of illness is real, having repercussions far deeper than we realize.

How many more high school shooting do we need in order to realize we're valuing the wrong things and failing our kids? When children don't get the love and attention they need, they shut down or act out. They can sense when mom and dad are unhappy, even when everyone is pretending things are fine. Self-worth grows strong in an environment of honesty and compassion. Self-worth gets damaged in an environment of lies and hostility.

What is a child supposed to do with feelings of confusion, neglect, and shame? Instead of listening to our kids, because they deserve our respect, we throw pills at them because we're too busy. Take this pill so you won't remember the past. Take this pill because you're not acting like everyone else. Take this pill to chase away the gloom. Take this pill when you can't sleep at night. Take this pill and everything will be alright.

With all of these pills "solving our problems," we have an excuse not to do the inner work. True healing comes from the inside. Happiness doesn't come from a bottle, and you'll never drink enough to drown your sorrow. Medication should be used in conjunction with cognitive behavioral therapy, so we can get to the root of the problem. We slap band-aids on deep wounds and pretend we don't see the blood. Medicating inner turmoil doesn't make it go away; it makes it worse.

Who wouldn't be depressed after receiving a cancer diagnosis and enduring the agony of treatment? I was lucky to escape with my breasts and ovaries. Many women aren't as lucky. The pink ribbon is a tiny reward for losing the parts of us that make us women. How do we stay strong when we're stripped of our strength? How do we not have animosity towards a medical system that leaves us scarred and broken? I feel depressed when I think about the cancer coming back. I feel depressed when I cave into peer pressure. Depression feels ubiquitous and unending. Let me out! Save me! Help me! I want to belong. Can I join your group?

If reading about cutting triggers you or causes euphoric recall, please skip the next few paragraphs. The few times I've self-harmed were attempts to release emotional pain; they were cries for help, not suicide attempts. Cutting is not the answer; it provides short-term relief from long-term pain.

The pain had been building up for several weeks. I was freaking out all the time. I began hitting my thighs with my fist whenever I did something wrong. I really hadn't done anything wrong. I was being hard on myself again, demanding perfection from an imperfect situation.

That night, I was sitting on the couch talking to my mom on the phone. We usually have good conversations, and she helps me get things figured out, but this time I didn't feel heard. I was upset with myself, because I was becoming dependent on her again. I felt trapped like I was going to burst. After we ended our phone call, I ran into the kitchen, opened the silverware drawer, grabbed the small knife I use to slice my banana in the morning, and started grinding on my inner forearm between my wrist and elbow, making two-inch slices.

I must've been dissociating because it didn't hurt, even though I was drawing blood. I felt some relief, yet it was short-lived, because the cuts were bleeding and they hurt. It was summer time; I had to wear short sleeves and let people see the cuts. This is what pain looks like when you don't let it out in appropriate doses. It shouldn't have come to this, but it did. Hopefully, the next time the wind releases me, I won't go looking for my next tree. I will enjoy my freedom.

※

I remember a text message my friend, Steve, sent to me a few months after treatment ended, "So, have you put all that cancer stuff behind you?"

At the time, "all that cancer stuff" was very much front and center; there was no way I could've answered, "Yes." I was at the beginning of my recovery feeling hopeful that things would get better. I had no idea I was going to go through the pain, fatigue, anxiety, and depression. I thought I'd recover much quicker than I did; I underestimated the possible repercussions of cancer treatment.

He was probably just making conversation and concerned about my well-being, yet his question struck a chord with me. The bitter part of me wanted to answer, "Oh yes, I've swept 'all that cancer stuff' under the rug, and it's business as usual. I'm going to be dealing with this for awhile; I guess you won't be a part of that."

Now that I have a few years of perspective, I could answer his text: "Yes, I'm trying to move forward and enjoy my life. Can you help me with that?"

I don't remember what my reply was. I probably listed my struggles. If only I had put "all that cancer stuff" behind me, I wouldn't be sitting here dragging myself through it. He knew my cancer experience was going to have a significant impact on me. He was worried that I'd be lost forever.

If only I had let someone help me, perhaps my recovery would've gone smoother. I can't change the past; I can make better choices now. His question is a good example of how our society is uncomfortable with illness and death, rushing people through their healing and grieving process.

How do we use our cancer experience as a catalyst for change, rather than a crutch to stay sick? How do we turn post-traumatic stress into growth? It takes hard work to get well, a sincere desire to rejoin the world, and an honest attempt at forgiveness. We can't push people away, because healing doesn't happen in isolation. I know the depths of despair and the strength of determination. I know the bitterness of defeat and the resilience of spirit. I know the beauty of nature and the necessity of laughter.

My breakthrough came when I decided to be a proud survivor instead of an angry victim. I heard a voice telling me everything was going to be okay. When I'm expressing my authentic self and reaching for my highest good, the Universe opens doors for me. I make it sound easy, but I haven't made it easy on myself. My healing journey forced me to slow down and take care of myself, the person I always put last; the person who needed my love the most.

There's a lesson in the pain if we're brave enough to look for it. One day, I heard a knock on the front door. When I went to answer it, I found a brown box sitting on the porch. The sun moved out from behind the clouds, causing the box to glisten like liquid gold. I blinked my eyes in disbelief. I looked up and down the street for the delivery truck. He must've sped away. The label was addressed to me. I brought the box inside and sat it on the kitchen table. I used scissors to slice the packing tape. The box was empty except for a small, pink envelope. Inside the envelop was a hand-written note: "When you love yourself, the darkness disappears." Can it really be that easy? Yes, self-love is the path to health and happiness.

My mom said to me one day, "You're writing a self-help book." I looked around my room at all of the motivational quotes and pictures. I'm smart, but I'm always the last one to get the joke. I've been studying this stuff for years, immersing myself in the healing power of positive thinking. Inspiration has become my life whether I like it or not, and whether it's cool or not; it's the healthy part of me. There was a time in my life when I thought self-help literature was silly, but then my life changed, and I had to choose the light.

In October of 2015, my brother, David, and sister-in-law, Kristine, who live in Utah, came home to Ohio for a visit. I finally met my seven-month-old niece, Emma. She's adorable, energetic, and very perceptive. She's a happy baby. We went out for dinner the last night they were in town.

The waitress had an interesting tattoo on her arm. I was sitting at the end of the booth, so I noticed it when she delivered the meals.

"What does your tattoo say?" I asked.

She showed me her arm. *Only God can judge me.*

Wow! Powerful words. Depression is often the result of judging ourselves without mercy, and allowing the judgment of others to bring us down. I think God is a kind judge, giving us credit when our intentions are pure and forgiving us when we're led astray.

CHAPTER SIX

Walking the Labyrinth

I still have days when I'm not proud of my recovery. My friends wonder if they'll ever see me again. I was diagnosed with breast cancer at an age when most women are getting married and having children. Why my life took the path it did, I'll never know for sure. At the end of the day, my theories don't keep me warm. I have to trust that this experience will lead me to something better—a new friend, a new outlook, a new purpose, a new adventure, a new life.

And yet, I'm afraid of a recurrence because I'm not choosing health every day. I'm still feeding the cancer with sugar, stress, and sadness. My cells want to be nourished with love, light, and laughter. There's a part of me that's given up. Some days, I don't want to live. I'm tired of fighting. I'm worried the darkness will overpower the light, and chaos will grow in strength. Death laughed in my face, and Light wouldn't take me. I still have lessons to learn, like how to love myself as much as God does. I have to choose the light because darkness + darkness = more darkness.

I fought fire with fire. And then I wondered what would've happened if I had chosen peace? What if I had stopped after the lumpectomy and refused treatment? Would I still be here today to ask my silly questions? Did standard treatment kill the microscopic cancer cells or were they just put to sleep? I probably sound like an ungrateful lunatic to knock treatment and voice my frustration. Perhaps, I am.

I've heard of spontaneous remission and miracle cures. Which leads me to ask: Can the mind heal the body? Can we cure cancer with natural remedies? Are alternative treatments reliable? Holistic healing is less damaging, but is it as effective? I didn't have enough faith or courage to find out. It would've made me responsible for my life. I would've had to heal myself from the inside out. Now, I'm going to do whatever it takes to stay alive. Perhaps, the best course of action is a combination of standard and holistic.

Do I still want a cigarette? Sure. I smoked a pack-a-day for three years. Cigarettes gave me a sense of comfort and security, which was in equal measures harmful and addicting. Am I going to smoke a cigarette? No. My drive to be healthy is stronger than my drive to be sick. I stopped smoking cigarettes in 2008. I make a daily choice to stay sober. I avoid the potholes. I walk down a different street. There's nothing good about addiction. There's no reason to give your power away, ever.

Being disconnected from my needs made it easy for me to help others and put myself last. I thought I was being a good person to go without what I needed. It took not having anything to give for me to stop giving it away. It shouldn't have come to that. I should've respected myself enough not to let others disrespect me. I shouldn't have chased every boy in town looking for love and approval. I shouldn't have worked myself to death at a job that wasn't fulfilling to me. I should've given myself a break before the Universe did.

We need to trust our gut instinct when something doesn't feel right, whether it's a job, city, career, house, relationship, or even a sweater; we always know. It's much harder to admit, "Hey, I need to get the hell out of here. This is not where I want to be. I've made the wrong choice, and I need to change course." Honesty is a better course of action than staying stuck. Look at the things you complain about. Are they things you've chosen? Are they things you can change?

It wasn't until I lost my boyfriend, dad, health, hair, job, and peace of mind that I figured out what really matters and what never did. The things I took for granted were taken from me. I was careless and flippant. God doesn't like to be mocked. Even beautiful things become ugly if we don't take care of them.

I'm saddened by the fact that so many people are diagnosed with cancer. The more we can tell the truth about our experience, the more we'll help others. When we stop pretending things are fine, we can experience true healing and transformation. I have to wear my heart on my sleeve and be bulletproof to criticism, which isn't an easy thing to do. This is my journey home, back to the source of everything which is love.

Life becomes an ecstatic dance when you discover your soul calling. The Universe will not lead you astray. Trust what brings you joy. The real work is effortless. I thought I had to struggle and manipulate. My pushy ego tried to take what wasn't mine. When we're walking the wrong path, we have to force things to happen. When we're on the right path, everything comes into focus and makes sense.

The poet Rainer Maria Rilke wrote, "We must trust in what is difficult." He doesn't mean suffering and heartbreak, although great art often arises from that place. He means stretching past our comfort zone and learning new things. Change is difficult because we're creatures of habit. We have to develop discipline and appreciate the stillness. We have to push ourselves so that we are experiencing personal growth. We also have to pause and reflect on our accomplishments.

My graduate school was a little different. First of all, it was located in Santa Fe, New Mexico, the land of enchantment. Secondly, it offered art therapy and counseling degrees where we were expected to heal our wounds and become good therapists. So, it wasn't surprising that my Archetypal Psychology class made mandalas and took a field trip to a park down the street where we walked a man-made labyrinth. The experience has always stuck with me. My teacher planted a seed that took me many years to understand.

The cancer experience, like walking the labyrinth, is a journey with many twists and turns, but the way in and the way out are the same path. When it comes to healing, there are no shortcuts. We journey within so that we can straighten out the knots, speak kindly to our inner child, and usher them out of hiding. It's similar to a meditation practice, we get in touch with the place inside of us that is calm and balanced. When we return to the world, we're stronger, wiser, and able to deal with challenges.

PART II

LESSONS I'VE LEARNED

CHAPTER ONE

Slow Down

Like many cancer survivors, I feel compelled to find meaning in my experience. On good days, I can tie this into a pretty bow. On bad days, I get out the scissors and cut the ribbon to shreds. I think the real recovery begins when we switch our question from, "Why did this happen to me?" to "What can I learn from this?"

I've learned how to slow down and appreciate the beauty around me. I've learned that forgiveness weighs less than a grudge. I've spent the last five years trying to tell my story, always finding an excuse not to be brave enough. Writing about my experience has kept me going, and it's wearing me out. I need to move onto the next chapter of my life. I have novels to write, affirmation cards to make, adventures to take, and people to love.

It's important to learn as much as we can about cancer, because knowledge is power. We can't put up a strong fight if we're uneducated and running scared. How do you rebuild your life after everything falls apart? Very carefully. You'll need a strong foundation, optimism, faith, determination, and a support system. Trying to do it all on your own is not going to be easy; I know because I've tried. There's nothing wrong with needing help, even God gets help from the angels.

How did I get cancer? What caused my cells to divide abnormally and form a malignant tumor? There are many theories of disease to choose from. I can blame it on my genes, environment, emotional health, or soul purpose. Everything in the Universe is interconnected, so it'd be naïve to choose just one cause. Since our thoughts create our reality, it'd be arrogant not to take personal responsibility. Whatever is in the mind will manifest itself in the body. Our unresolved emotional issues will get played out in some form of illness or drama. Even if you don't believe in the soul, it'd be narrow-minded to eliminate the possibility.

I believe disease is caused by a combination of nature, nurture, and spirituality. Our genes + our environment + our soul's mission = what happens to us. There are many forces at work, and we cannot comprehend them all. We have free will to change the course of events, and there's a strong probability we're headed for a certain destiny. Our mental, physical, and emotional health is directly related to our thoughts, behaviors, and feelings. We have the power to restore balance and harmony.

I'm like my grandma, Mary, stubborn as hell with a big heart; it takes a lot to knock us down. Mary is 89 years old; her hair is still reddish brown because the gray hair knows better. She asks me, "How are you, Ladybug?" It's one of my favorite things because she really wants to know. She works crossword puzzles and will pick up every leaf in her yard if you let her. She has dementia now. She can't remember what she ate for lunch, but she can tell you about the love she had for my grandpa like it was yesterday.

At first, my recovery was a never-ending mission to get my old normal back. I thought if I exercised enough or gave it more time, I could magically heal the damage that had been done. I was naïve about chemotherapy and radiation, thinking myself young and resilient enough to escape its toxicity. I jumped onto the pink ribbon bandwagon and didn't look back until it was too late. The problem with fighting is that once you start it's hard to stop. I was determined to be a good patient and kick cancer's ass. It never dawned on me that I might not be standing in the final round.

When my physical endurance reached a plateau, light years behind my pre-cancer self, I decided to be okay with this because at least I wasn't still bed-ridden, leaking spinal fluid. When the emotional devastation caught up with me, I experienced panic attacks and post-traumatic stress disorder. Cancer treatment also exacerbated my obsessive-compulsive disorder. The only thing that grew stronger was my faith in God and the angels. Nevertheless, I was a disgruntled survivor. I couldn't reconcile in my mind how something could help me and hurt me at the same time. I took the treatment to live, and it felt like I had died. I couldn't move on. I couldn't let it go.

Stuck in the victim role, unable to find the silver lining, the days blurred together. I went to doctor after doctor (neurologist, cardiologist, rheumatologist, and otolaryngologist), asking them to fix what the treatment broke. My body still functioned in the normal range, but the low end felt completely different from the high end, and all they could offer me was medication, which meant more side effects. I had punished myself enough. It was time to stop fighting and let my poor, wounded body heal itself.

My new normal made me resent the treatment that had saved my life. It didn't matter how bad I felt; I had to take responsibility for my choices. It's taken me a long time to understand why acceptance is the last stage of grief. I had to go through denial, anger, bargaining, and depression to properly mourn my losses. I could then move forward with a healthy perspective of wisdom and compassion.

It was time to forgive and forget, which is easier said than done. I didn't ask about the long-term side effects, and even if I had it probably wouldn't have made a difference; I wanted the reassurance that came with standard treatment. Unfortunately, with cancer there are no guarantees, and the possibility of recurrence always lurks in the shadows.

I put on my brave face to get through treatment and then I fell apart. I thought I was being punished for something: being angry at my father, cheating on my boyfriend, not petting enough cute puppies. Dear God, if you fix this mess, I promise to be a better person. It's taken me a long time to develop a rational perspective on the situation.

Getting cancer made me feel like I was being tested by the Universe. I remember taking tests in school. When I learned the material, the test was easy. When I memorized the material, I no idea what to write for the essay question.

Let's test your ability to see cancer as a gift. What lesson was the illness trying to teach you? Self-love. Are you treating yourself with loving kindness? I'm trying.

Have you gotten your priorities in order? For the most part.

What positive qualities have you developed? A sense of humor.

Are you living your life in a way that is meaningful to you? I'm being creative.

Have you found the silver lining? I'm grateful to be alive. I know what's important and what never was. Time is of the essence, and we have plenty of time. The further I got away from my path, the louder God had to yell. Now, I slow down and listen for the whispers.

Grade: A+

CHAPTER TWO

Speak Up

When I was young, I played soccer and tee ball. I also took ballet and gymnastics lessons. When it came time for me to focus on one sport, there was no doubt in my mind which one was my favorite: soccer. As I grew older, I played on select teams traveling to weekend tournaments. I always wore my tournament t-shirt to school because I was proud of my team. I also played volleyball and basketball, but they paled in comparison.

In high school, I made the varsity soccer team as a freshman, starting as center forward. This was a big deal and my confidence was sky-high. I was also dating a senior named Wes. And then the summer before my junior year, I had a bit of an accident. I pooped my pants during one of my select soccer practices. I had eaten a bowl of chili before practice. Luckily, I was wearing bicycle shorts underneath my soccer shorts and one of my teammates lived nearby, so I was able to go to her house to clean up a bit. I'm sure her mom didn't appreciate the mess I left in her bathroom.

I was more concerned with getting back to practice, because I didn't want to get in trouble. I continued practicing even though gnats were attracted to the smell and kept landing on my shin guards. Some of my teammates realized what happened and laughed at me. I should've told my coach what happened, sat out, and waited for my dad to return to pick me up. Instead, my people-pleaser personality followed the rules and pretended everything was okay.

Although the odds of having another accident were slim-to-none, I worried it would happen again. My mind was preoccupied with thoughts of whether I needed to go to the bathroom or not, which only made matters worse. I wouldn't eat anything three hours before a game or practice, so there wouldn't be anything in my stomach.

I lost my focus and competitive edge. I no longer enjoyed playing soccer. Everyone noticed the change, and I quit after senior year. Instead of facing my fears, I became a quitter. Soccer had been my life, my source of confidence, and to go without it felt strange. My family assumed I'd play in college, and I guess that was the game plan. My dad took me to visit several colleges, but I knew without a doubt I couldn't play anymore. I don't know who I disappointed more: him or me.

Looking back, not only was soccer healthy for me physically, it taught me something about how to fight cancer. How do you prepare for the big game? In soccer, we jogged around the field warming our muscles, getting touches on the ball, taking shots on goal while trying to intimidate the other team. We looked sharp in our blue-and-white-checkered uniforms. We put our hair in ponytails or French braids.

We waved to our moms sitting in their lawn chairs, interrupting their chit-chat. They were always there cheering us on, in the winter covered up in blankets, and in the summer sweating with the rest of us. Our dads stood on the sidelines following the action, ready to yell at the referee over a bad call.

I never sat the bench. I was one of the best players on the team. I was aggressive, arrogant, fearless, a force to be reckoned with, and a goalie's worst nightmare. I had a natural athletic ability that made playing sports fun.

My team formed a huddle, clasping our hands together at the center. My coach gave a pep talk that ended with a loud cheer. We ran onto the field and got into our positions. The referee started his stopwatch and blew the whistle. Game on!

What's the warm-up for cancer treatment? Get a good night sleep and eat a healthy breakfast. Pack a small bag with comfort items: pen, journal, book, music, snack, and sweatshirt. Write down questions to ask your doctor. Bring your laptop to blog, catch up on email, or watch videos. Sometimes, the pre-meds put me to sleep, so I didn't need all the things I brought! Arrive early for your appointments so you can fill out paperwork.

When a doctor gives you a knowing look and says, "You have about a month before treatment starts," what they really mean is this: the person you are now, how great you feel; all those warm and fuzzy feelings are probably going to go out the window. You'd better go and do some wild, crazy things.

Don't wait until you're faced with death to appreciate life. Start living now. Send an email to the guy you like. What's the worst thing that can happen? He doesn't email you back. His loss! The cool shirt you're saving for a special occasion? Wear it today.

Don't prepare for the bad times. Well, prepare a little. Just make sure you drink that margarita, put on your fancy clothes to go dancing with your friends, because a month from now those memories will pull you through the dark days and even darker nights. You have a long road ahead of you; begin the journey with some good memories.

Remember, you are not your hair. If you need hair, buy a wig. If you don't want a wig, buy a hat or scarf. If you don't need hair, rock the bald-is-beautiful look. As if you don't feel bad enough already, now your vanity will be tested. At least you don't have to buy shampoo or fix your hair for awhile. Look on the bright side!

Develop cancer teammates. Get to know the patients sitting next to you, as they can relate to what you're going through. The first time you get treatment can feel overwhelming, because you don't know what to expect. Once you get the routine down and get to know the nurses, you'll feel much better. You'll learn as you go and find strength you never knew you had.

Halftime is when the coach changes strategy based on what's not working. Do we need a stronger offense or defense? Are the set plays working? Do we need to change our game plan? Halftime is when you take a breather and get your second wind. Treat yourself to a refreshing beverage and snack. Talk with your teammates about your hopes, dreams, and plans for the future.

Imagine yourself scoring a goal in the second half, then doing a victory dance by the corner flag. Visualize the scoreboard showing your team as the winner. The cheerleaders are rallying you to victory. H-U-S-T-L-E! You can do it. Hang in there. You're doing great! You're the courageous one, an inspiration to the spectators.

Check in with your body. How are you feeling? Tell your doctor your symptoms. You don't have to be the heroine. Fighting the good fight sometimes means walking away. Listen to your intuition. Your body knows when enough is enough. Don't make choices from a place of fear or bravado.

There are many ways to fight cancer. Be your own advocate. Doctors are not mind readers. If something doesn't feel right, let them know. You don't have to suffer in silence. The side effects are not to be taken lightly; they can cause permanent damage. Don't underestimate the repercussions of cancer treatment. Ask questions. Get answers. Be a bad patient. This is your life. You can slow down and sit the bench. The finish line will be there tomorrow.

I made a list for you with some important things I've learned along the way.

My Ten Little Gems of Wisdom

1. A strong person asks for help.
2. We change when we're ready to change.
3. Aim for good enough. Perfection is a trap.
4. Every day is a gift. Don't take it for granted.
5. There's always an angel nearby cheering for you.
6. It's easier to move forward if you leave the past behind.
7. If you need to break something, start with your bad habits.
8. The reason we're here is to love, laugh, and learn.
9. If they're calling you crazy, you're on the right track.
10. It doesn't matter if everyone else doubts your ability; it only matters if you join them.

CHAPTER THREE

Choose Health

Have you ever thought to yourself, how did I get here? I please everyone but myself. My clothes are threadbare. I don't feel good. I'm all alone. Nobody loves me. My job is boring. My kids won't listen to me. The house is a wreck. I can't pay the bills. I smile at the neighbors even though I'm dying inside. Pour me another drink, we're going to have some fun tonight. I'm burning the candle at both ends to prove I'm good enough.

Is he ever going to email me back? I see three more gray hairs. I used to be happy and funny and beautiful. I'm getting fat. I don't feel like exercising. I don't have time to fix healthy meals. Let's go through the drive thru. I've got nothing left to lose. I can take medication when I get sick. Turn on the television, I need to unwind.

That reel of tape gets us nowhere because it's filled with negativity. Negativity gains momentum, gathers troops, spreads rumors, and wreaks havoc in our bodies. At least we're being honest about how bad things are, but we aren't making changes.

We become sick when we stop choosing health. Well, duh! If it's so obvious, then why are we struggling with addiction, depression, obesity, and spiritual emptiness? Oftentimes, we deny the mind-body-spirit connection because that would make us responsible for our health. It's much easier to blame something outside of ourselves, but the funny thing is, we put that stuff there, too.

Seeking solutions is a much better use of our time than bitching and complaining. The way to get unstuck is to think more positively. Even if the positive thoughts are a million miles away from where we actually are, at least we're taking control of our mental focus. Eventually, we'll get there. There are so many other things to be than miserable. There are so many ways to let our light shine.

I know how scary it is to take a leap of faith. When the man of my dreams offered me the world, instead of graciously accepting and thanking my lucky stars, I told him I just wanted to be friends. In those moments, when we're on the precipice of change, the best thing to do is slow down, take a deep breath, and tell the truth. "I want to walk toward you, but there isn't any ground to walk on. I'm scared of what you're offering me because it's everything I've ever wanted. Can you help me?" And he probably would've said something like, "I'll carry you until you find your footing. I'm scared too, but I'm willing to take a chance."

He would've challenged me to grow and become a better person. My dad had just died, and I was dealing with that. *That's a poor excuse for being afraid of happiness.* I think I got cancer because I pushed love away. I'm afraid it could happen again. I wasn't ready to change back then, but I ended up changing anyway. It's funny how our lives come full circle, and we arrive back where we started much older and wiser. Make it easy on yourself; don't get there kicking and screaming or filled with regret.

Recovery is a time to recuperate and get your strength back. We have to acknowledge, rather than minimize, what we've been through. The cancer experience changes you; the key is to have it change you for the better. It's hard not to be bitter about chronic pain and fatigue. I take the good with the bad and find a reason to laugh. Some days this is easier than others.

When I went for my oncology check-ups, I noticed how some of the patients I'd gone through treatment with weren't struggling. Leave it to my competitive nature to compare myself and come up short. Maybe they were struggling, but I couldn't see it. Like me, they tried to make a good impression—the bravest of the brave. Next time, I'll ask them instead of making assumptions. Maybe they were afraid to reach out, too.

CHAPTER FOUR

Compassion

I'm an Adult Child of an Alcoholic (ACoA.) I grew up in an environment that was at times unpredictable and chaotic. When I read the list of characteristics, I'm blown away because it describes many of my core issues: need for control, all-or-none thinking, fear of abandonment, low self-esteem, approval seeker, extreme loyalty, overly responsible, avoids feelings, has difficulty following through, creates drama, neglects needs, and rescues others.

I often guess at normal behavior and true intimacy. I learned the unspoken rules, "don't talk, don't trust, and don't feel," which maintain the addict's ability to use by controlling the emotional climate of the household. It's important to know how we were affected, not to place blame, so we can recognize our patterns and make healthier choices in the future.

I was an expert at holding grudges, having carried one for years against my father for being an alcoholic. After his death, I realized he had a serious addiction, and it was my animosity that strained our relationship. I'm finally learning how to see the past through the eyes of an adult rather than a hurt child. It doesn't bring my dad back or the years I lost being angry. My father was more than his addiction, and I am more than my disorders. We developed maladaptive coping mechanisms to deal with life stressors.

I've begged and pleaded for someone to love me when I didn't love myself. I appeared anxious and desperate, which aren't attractive qualities. The world mirrored back to me exactly what I thought. No wonder I felt miserable. I gave my power away, thinking I was too strong. Instead of embracing my freedom, I walked back into the prison. Instead of exploring my creative side, I put my paints into a box for safekeeping.

When you love yourself and have strong boundaries, you can give and take in equal measures. You won't let yourself get stripped bare of all you possess. When you have nothing left to lose, that's when you lose it all. The Universe wants you to be happy, I really believe this, and you can only mess up for so long, remember that.

When I was a teenager, I doubted my beauty and strength. When chemotherapy took my hair and energy, I had no choice but to look at myself with compassion. The people in my life never stopped loving me, and they don't need me to become someone else. They love me for who I am. They just want to see me and know that I'm okay. I thought I had to be perfect to be loved. Nobody is perfect. Nobody has the right answer.

We need to look at how we're living our lives. When we're constantly on the go, we neglect the necessary downtime to pause and reflect. Our inner work is just as important as our outer work. When we discover our soul purpose, it adds depth and meaning to our lives. Love makes us feel wealthy, even if we're struggling to make ends meet. Without a strong spiritual core, it's too easy to be distracted by the noise.

It's no wonder Americans are stereotyped as lazy, ignorant, and rude. We spend our time chasing fads, idolizing celebrities, worshiping wealth, and glorifying war. We become disconnected from our heart source. We know it's wrong, but we don't know how to make it right. We follow the crowd at the expense of our dreams. In our struggle to have more, we actually have less. The economic debt is a distraction from the real problem—our spiritual debt.

Our cells are listening intently for direction and feeling profoundly; they create with the tools they're given. A fear-based mentality creates a very different environment than a love-based mentality. When we choose fear, we produce an oppressive situation. We believe the lies and dim our light. We stop trusting ourselves. We shame others who are having a difficult time. We eat dinner with the bullies.

When we choose love, we can dance with the wild things. The wild things have vitality and wisdom to share for those who are listening. Love writes about a future we could have if we dare to dream. Fear convinces us we'll never amount to much. Love fights with integrity and grace. Fear fights with ignorance and malice. Love creates beautiful sunsets. Fear prevents miracles from occurring.

How do we align with the divine and reconnect with our spiritual source? Turn off the television, read more books, listen to music, spend time in nature, or start a meditation practice. Stop complaining and taking everything for granted. Realize you're capable of greatness. Rest when it's time to rest; work when it's time to work. Have faith that the angels will guide and protect you. Seasons change and wounds heal. We breathe deeply and give thanks.

At first, developing a self-care routine can feel selfish or weird, because we're used to helping others. Most of the time, they didn't need our help; we were the ones that needed help. Now that we're adults, we can get our needs met. We aren't at the mercy of our parents anymore. They did the best job they knew how to do.

We can take a personal inventory and ask the hard questions. What areas of my life need improvement? What is/isn't working? What small changes can I make? What is my next right action? What would love do now? What would my best friend tell me?

I made another list with ten awesome ways to be good to you.

How To Treat Yourself With Loving Kindness

1. Get enough sleep so that you feel rested.
2. Create healthy meal plans for the week.
3. Start an exercise routine that you enjoy.
4. Write in your gratitude journal every day.
5. Plan a family vacation or road trip with friends.
6. Watch your favorite movie in your pajamas.
7. Buy yourself something special like flowers or shoes.
8. Schedule a haircut, manicure, pedicure, or massage.
9. Go to an art museum or amusement park.
10. Sign up for a class you've always wanted to take.

CHAPTER FIVE

Self-Acceptance

When I was a little girl, I felt rich. I had a desk full of pens, markers, paper, glitter, stickers, stamps, and watercolors. What more could a girl ask for? Art making was where I expressed my emotions best. If I had realized that sooner, I would've spent more time processing things through art. It wasn't until college that I discovered my love for painting. Hanging out with art crowd made me feel like I had a new set of teammates.

My first art experience came from my next door neighbor, an elderly lady named Lil. She gave me acrylic painting lessons on flowers and landscapes. She taught me how to mix colors and wash out my brushes. My dad gave me a five-dollar bill to pay Lil for each lesson. It was very quiet at her house and, like my dad, she smoked cigarettes. She painted a basic outline and then I colored in the rest. When I got home, my dad would frame and hang the painting like it was really something special.

Growing up, my mom made good dinners, but I was a picky eater, hiding pieces of broccoli and pork chop in my napkin so I could leave the dinner table. My favorite meal was when we made pizzas. My brother and I went sled riding in the winter and watched fireworks in the summer. We played cards and board games. We ran around the yard catching lightning bugs in mason jars. We rode our bikes to the corner store to buy penny candy. We went on family vacations. We had lots of friends. Life was good.

I shied away from taking art classes in high school because I didn't have the natural ability to consider myself an artist. I was in the concert band and theater group. I liked fashion and jewelry. I was muscular from playing soccer and weighed about 135 pounds. In college, I lost about ten pounds; still in the healthy range for my five-foot-seven-inch small frame. In graduate school, life got even more chaotic, and I lost another ten pounds, but being at 115 didn't feel so good; I often felt lightheaded.

I was wearing a size zero, and for some reason it felt like an achievement to be that thin. Maybe now I'm okay, loveable, worthy, and amazing. If I look like the model on the cover of the glossy magazine, I'll be happy, right?

Being a certain size didn't solve my problems or bring me self-acceptance. If anything, it made everything worse. I was neglecting my mind, body, and spirit. Instead of enjoying food, I had a love-hate relationship with it. The real me was disappearing as I chased after the things I thought would make me happy.

I went to Butler University in Indianapolis, Indiana, my freshman year because my boyfriend, Ian, also got accepted there. Instead of branching out, we clung together and missed out on some of the typical college experiences. Without realizing it, my experience with restricting food planted the seed for an eating disorder.

I wasn't trying to lose weight back then; I was trying to prevent another accident. This was before eating disorders were rampant and popular. I'd only seen one documentary about a gymnast who nearly starved herself to death.

My boyfriend and I had fun going to bookstores, restaurants, and music concerts. Butler was a great college, but we were looking for something different, and we found it at Naropa University, the only Buddhist-inspired accredited college in North America. Ian wanted to attend the Jack Kerouac writing program. I threw together a portfolio of oil pastel pictures and applied for the Visual Art program, having never taken a real art class.

Luckily, we were both accepted. We begged our families to let us go because we were determined to follow our hearts and live our dreams. They let us go! We moved to Boulder, Colorado with our thrift store clothes, youthful exuberance, and his ten boxes of books. When I saw the Flatirons, the beautiful mountain range, my jaw hit the floor of our Budget rental van; it was like we'd found the magic city.

My art teachers encouraged creative self-expression, so I didn't feel hindered by my lack of skill. There was something so satisfying about abstract painting—I could make a mess. I didn't have to be perfect. I was in control of the lines and shapes. I lost track of time when I painted. I released my inner turmoil with black and red paint.

We graduated in 2000, and moved home because we missed our

families. The rent was getting expensive, too. I didn't want to leave because I liked living out there; open space is good for the soul.

Three years later, I drove all the way to Santa Fe, New Mexico (in two days) by myself to start graduate school. Although I was trying to be independent, the city overwhelmed me. A week later, I called my boyfriend asking him for help. Ian drove out there, and we got an apartment together near school. He got a full-time job, and I was busy with school. But things were different this time. Maybe we were growing apart.

I met a guy that I liked. I thought the grass was greener on the other side. It was more like a yard full of rocks. Ian and I broke up, and he moved back home. I was left with my own anger and arrogance. Looking back, I'd tell myself, "Don't work out your issues like that. Don't throw away true love for a moment of nothingness." Unfortunately, life doesn't work that way. We do stupid things and have to learn from our mistakes.

My family flew out to attend my graduation ceremony. We had a good time going to the tourist attractions and local restaurants. We visited art museums, historic chapels, the plaza, and Canyon Road. We hiked Bandeleir National Monument. It was their second visit, but this time my dad wasn't feeling so good.

I wasn't doing so well, either. In my graduation pictures, I look frighteningly thin. I weighed about 108 pounds which was the lowest I'd ever been. I didn't know how I was going to use my art therapy degree; I had more issues than *National Geographic*. I wasn't ready to be an art therapist. My artwork was dark and dreary.

Even though I completed my coursework, I hadn't resolved my issues. I knew my emotional baggage would prevent me from being a good therapist. I made the right decision and spent more time getting life experience. I wondered if I'd ever make happy pictures and step into my role as a healer.

No matter what I did, my repressed anger and low self-esteem usually got in the way. Food was the one thing I could control because my life was not my own. I focused on pleasing others and lost my identity in the process. It took getting cancer to make me heal my wounds and develop self-compassion. My dad loved me. His addiction to alcohol had nothing to do with me, and it wasn't my job to save him.

When I restricted food, I didn't count calories. I controlled my portion sizes and chewed very slowly. I didn't want to feel full. I didn't want to *feel*. Usually, I hadn't eaten enough and felt hungry soon after, which mirrored my hunger for love and affection. I always saved room for dessert, being comforted by sugary sweets: ice cream and cookies. I knew the dessert would never abandon me.

There's a certain weight our bodies like to be at, which is different for everyone because it's based on height and frame. When I'm at my optimum weight, I feel good and have an abundance of energy. Food is fuel and nourishment; it's a gift we give ourselves. Now, I look forward to eating delicious meals with my friends and family.

We are more than the numbers on our jeans, the color of our eye shadow, or the length of our hair. We are complicated creatures who try too hard, do too much, and are often misunderstood. We can appreciate our femininity and realize it is our true power. We can be like the goddesses who are revered for being strong.

The longer I stayed isolated, the worse I became. As soon as I reached out, I made some new friends and they encouraged me. I don't know what I was so worried about? I am a good writer and my message is important. Real friends push you to do your best and are happy when you succeed. Fake friends point out your flaws and bring you down.

Arriving at self-acceptance doesn't happen overnight, or maybe it does. I woke up one day and realized I am a good person. I never needed their permission or validation. I'm the only one who knows what I need and how I feel. I'm going to do things that make me happy, even if I disappoint someone else. Life is too short to listen to other people's nonsense, or worry about superficial things. We are good enough; the world tries to convince us otherwise.

CHAPTER SIX

Ending Well

Your team is leading two-to-one in the final minutes of the game. The crowd is standing in anticipation and cheering loudly. The other team is trying to tie the score. They take one last shot on goal; it goes wide, and the referee blows his whistle. Game over! Shake the other team's hand. Good game. Good game.

You've finished treatment. Now what? Hopefully, you'll experience a smooth transition into "life after cancer." To be on the safe side, prepare for some rainy weather and a few alligators in the pond. You've fought hard; give yourself time to recuperate. The people who'll understand what you've been through are your fellow survivors. You can share remedies for dealing with lingering side effects.

What I noticed is my role switched from patient to survivor, and my doctors moved on to the next scared patient. Instead of having a calendar filled with doctor appointments, I had time to go places and do fun things. I wish I'd gotten rid of everything associated with treatment: clothes, hats, bed sheets, and my victim mentality. I struggled with my post-cancer identity. I didn't feel like the old me. I balked at my new normal thinking it wasn't good enough. I should've been grateful to be alive.

I stayed stuck because there wasn't enough forward momentum. I had unhealthy assumptions about being sick. It put me in the spotlight, but it was a negative spotlight. I don't have to get sick to be cared for and loved. I don't have to wait for my body to collapse to take a break. I don't have to be superwoman. I can be loved for who I am, because who I am is pretty darn amazing! And most days, I am superwoman.

Being honest about how we're feeling is the first step towards healing. If we build walls to keep people out, eventually we'll succeed. I think people want to help, they just don't know how. We can tell them, "This is what I'm going through; this is how you can help me." Sometimes, we need a break from cancer, a mental reprieve, an emotional vacation. Laughter is the best medicine, because it causes our cells to dance with joy.

Everybody is ready to celebrate your victory but you still feel like slime on the bottom of the ocean. I know how you feel. I tried to step back in line, but the line was gone. I tried to hop on board, but the train had already left the station. I waited for the next train which never came. You can't pick up where you left off; at least I couldn't.

I heard stories about good restaurants and funny movies. Everyone was whistling a happy tune while my iPod shuffled the sad songs. I was devastated because my body was destroyed. Everything that needed to be done accumulated in piles around me. I went from being successful and confident to being overwhelmed and depressed.

I don't know how I survived the whole ordeal. I don't know how anyone does. I believe there is a power greater than myself that saved me, because I still have work to do. I believe love is the answer, love like there's no tomorrow. Hope floats a sinking ship, and in the darkest hour comes the light. It's easier to heal a small wound than one that's been festering for years. If we don't face our demons, our demons will face us. It takes more energy to numb and run than it does to breathe and release.

If you're struggling with the emotional fallout of cancer treatment, see a therapist. It's quite possible your caregivers have compassion fatigue, and you'll benefit more from outside support. Even though we've streamlined nearly everything in our lives, we can't hurry the healing or grieving process.

Don't underestimate what you've been through or let someone else minimize your experience. You are special. What you went through was horrible. You fought the good fight and deserve to celebrate. It's normal to feel like a changed person. Life looked completely different to me after treatment. Please don't get lost in your sadness like I did. There's a whole world out there waiting for your contribution.

They say the location of the tumor represents the lesson you need to learn. For me, the breast represents nurturing and nourishment, things I still struggle with today. Why is it so difficult to be good to *me*? Why do I think it's acceptable to suffer?

A strong woman is able to surrender and receive. She doesn't hide in the tower brushing her long blonde hair. She makes it easy, ha, not too easy. She meets him halfway. He can jump the moat and scale the drawbridge. Men are hardwired to be the protector. They want to help us; it makes them feel good. I was afraid I'd get hurt if I opened up, yet I got hurt anyway withholding affection. Mixed messages are confusing.

Did my journey end well? Yes, the things I used to reach for no longer interest me. Even though it feels like it's taken forever, my recovery has been successful. How do I know for sure? The darkness is gone. My wounds are healed. My artwork is filled with happiness and bright colors. My heart feels free to love again. Big sigh of relief.

This list brings together all the ideas we've covered thus far. Which step are you on? It's perfectly fine to bounce around the steps. Healing is a lifelong process, there will always be opportunities to do more work around self-love and forgiveness. We share our stories because it helps us put the pieces of the puzzle together. We can then be comforted by people who care and understand. Recovery can be a magical experience!

The Twelve Steps To A Successful Recovery

1. Tell your story.
2. Acknowledge the pain.
3. Practice compassion.
4. Extend forgiveness.
5. Heal your wounds.
6. Release the past.
7. Envision a new future.
8. Move in that direction.
9. Trust your intuition.
10. Follow your heart.
11. Shine your light.
12. Live your dreams

PART III:

ART THERAPY AND WRITING EXERCISES

Introduction

Do you remember my promise to offer you some creative tools to facilitate recovery? Well, here they are! Drawing on my art therapy background, I've chosen the eleven best exercises for healing. Some of them have been around for awhile; some of them are my brand new creations. I tweaked them so they'd apply to what we're doing: Strength Building For Survivors. Your mind, body, and spirit will thank you.

The exercises are merely starting points. Allow what needs to come out move through you. Give yourself permission to play. What's important is that you're able to express yourself and find strength in your creations. Beginning a journey of self-discovery is an amazing gift you have given to yourself. When you're ready, share your artwork and writing with your therapist, close friend, or family member.

Scribble Drawing

Materials: Drawing paper. Pen, markers, crayons, or colored pencils.

Instructions: Make a flowing, continuous line on your paper. Keep scribbling until you feel ready to stop. Next, color in the shapes formed from the lines. You will be able to create an abstract design or something representational. When you're finished, give your picture a title. Good work!

The scribble drawing was developed by art educator Florence Cane as a warm-up to help students build creative confidence. If you're having trouble being spontaneous, use your non-dominant hand and close your eyes while you're scribbling.

Emotions Color Wheel

Materials: Drawing paper. Pen, markers, crayons, or colored pencils. Notebook.

Instructions: Draw a large circle which takes up most of the paper. Divide the circle into eight parts using four lines. It will look like a pie chart.

Choose eight emotions. For example: anger, fear, sadness, happiness, anxiety, love, hope, guilt, grief, gratitude, regret, frustration, and loneliness.

Write one emotion above each piece of the pie.

Next, color in each section to represent that emotion. Use images, shapes, symbols, or words. The possibilities are endless!

Which emotions have you been feeling recently? Which emotions would you like to feel more often? What activities in your life generate positive emotions? How do you cope with difficult emotions? Answer these questions in your notebook.

Pivotal Moments

Materials: Drawing paper. Markers, crayons, or colored pencils. Pen and notebook.

Instructions: Create a timeline of your pivotal moments. Choose at least ten experiences. For example: birth, school, graduation, divorce, job promotion, relocation, sports, hobbies, vacations, relationships, illness, trauma, addiction, or loss of a loved one.

Sketch a small scene on your paper to represent each pivotal moment.

Answer these questions in your notebook: What are your favorite memories? What challenges have you faced? How have they shaped you into the person you are today? What lessons have you learned? What miracles have you experienced?

Which experiences on your timeline have a negative emotional charge which signifies you have healing to do regarding that event? Are you nursing resentment and need to practice forgiveness? What do you think your next pivotal moment will be?

Dear Cancer Letter

Materials: Pen and notebook.

Instructions: Are you a patient, survivor, caregiver, doctor, or nurse? Have you lost someone you loved to cancer? Write a letter expressing your honest feelings. See my example:

Dear Cancer,

You're an unwelcome visitor. Go back to where you came from and leave me alone. I have no use for you here. I don't want your lessons. I want to go back to sleep. You want me to cherish life, be brave, and fly free. I want these things, too. I'm not afraid because I can weather any storm. All my life, I've been collecting pieces of shelter in preparation. A part of me has always known.

There've been glimpses of the future. I'm the one who chose this path. I will make you my ally, as silly as that sounds, and befriend the very thing that caused me pain. I will not be like you and spread darkness. Your insults hurt my hurt. I have a higher calling; to show you how to love. I see you, I hear you. I know what you want. I'll admit my mistakes, my stupid careless ways.

I'm different now; you've changed me. I think twice before I act flippant and unkind. I created you from lifetimes of fear and self-doubt. Every time I swallowed my anger, numbed the pain, and denied my power, you grew stronger. You're all of my hurts rolled into one. You feed off my sadness and resentment. You think you're the one creating the rules. I think one of us knows the way out.

This is a battle for my soul. I don't have to hide my light because it shines too bright. I don't have to pretend everything is fine. I offer you love not to grow and hurt me, to heal and be gone. You're as stuck as I am, lost and alone, causing trouble for no reason at all. Step into the light; show me who you are. Tell me how you feel, and I won't laugh at you. I can love us well. I can heal us whole. This is my rebirth. This is my thank you.

Sincerely,
Julie

Strength Box

Materials: Shoebox-sized paper mache box, magazines, scissors, and double sided tape.

Instructions: What gives you strength? What does strength look like to you? How does strength feel? Cut out images from a magazine, and collage them onto the box. Find the letters STRENGTH BOX and make a label. Wonderful!

This is your special box to store: cards, photos, quotes, comics, poems, recipes, crystals, and lucky charms. Only include items that give you strength. Keep it nearby so you can add more items. Look through the box when you need a boost of confidence.

Flower Mandala

Materials: Drawing paper. Pen, markers, crayons, or colored pencils. Notebook.

Instructions: Draw a large circle on your paper. If you were a flower, what kind would you be? Sketch a flower inside of the circle to represent how you're feeling today. Sometimes, becoming something else gives us a safe way to voice our frustrations.

Let the flower image immerge naturally. Focus on your breath so that it becomes a meditative exercise, too. Mandala is a Sanskrit word meaning circle or completion. Mandalas represent the universe, wholeness, harmony, and spiritual journeys.

Answer these questions outside of the circle, or in your notebook:

What does the flower need? What would it say if it had a voice? Is the flower growing and blooming, or barely hanging on? It is brightly colored or faded from the sun? What do the colors you've chosen represent?

Make another picture tomorrow or next week. Did you notice any changes?

Create a series of flower mandalas to show your healing progress and personal transformation. Years from now, you'll be glad to have a visual diary of your recovery.

Stepping Stones

Materials: Drawing paper. Pen, markers, crayons, or colored pencils. Notebook.

Instructions: Have you ever crossed a creek by jumping onto different rocks? Have you ever walked on pretty, mosaic stepping stones in someone else's garden?

Draw at least five stepping stones to represent the steps you need to take to have a successful recovery. Where are the stones located: in a garden, city, or stream? Are they close together, far apart, sturdy, or wobbly? Which stepping stone are you on? Are you at the beginning of your recovery or near the end? Who are the people cheering you on?

Write an encouraging word or a phrase on each stone. Do some journaling about recovery in your notebook. Buy an inexpensive frame at your local craft store, and hang the picture in your home as a reminder of your healing path.

Vision Board

Materials: Drawing paper. Magazines, scissors, double sided tape or glue.

Instructions: Imagine you are living the life of your dreams. Where do you live? Who are you with? What is your career? How do you spend your free time? What adjectives would you use to describe your life? How is it different from the life you're living now?

Look through some magazines. Cut out images and words that represent your dream life. Tape or glue them to a piece of paper to create a vision board collage.

Hang the vision board in your office or bedroom. Light a candle and mediate on your future. The Universe is always listening. Our thoughts are very powerful. Whatever we think about, we bring about. Manifestation is the simple process of visualizing the life we want, and then taking steps to make it happen.

Visualization + Effort + Magic = Results.

Gratitude Jar

Materials: Large glass mason jar. Acrylic paint materials. Pen and slips of paper.

Instructions: Paint the jar using your favorite colors and design. Make a label or paint the words "Gratitude Jar" on the outside of the jar. Place the jar in a prominent location. Keep pens and pre-cut slips of paper lying next to it.

Write down one thing you're thankful for on a piece of paper, and put it in the jar. For example: My husband made me breakfast. I had a great day at the beach. I bought a new sweater. I'm making progress on my novel. I saw a beautiful dragonfly on my walk.

Make this a daily, weekly, or whenever you feel inspired activity.

If you want, ask your friends or family members to participate. At the end of the month, read them aloud as a group. Which one was your favorite? Which ones made you smile? Does this activity help you focus on the good things in your life?

Start each month with an empty jar and a full heart. If there are some you don't want to throw away, write the date on the back, and put them in your Strength Box.

Gratitude Journal

Materials: Journal and pen.

Instructions: The purpose of a gratitude journal is to look for the good and appreciate our blessings. Write in your journal around the same time each day or night, as this will help you develop a routine. It's important to vary this activity, so you don't get bored.

Here are some ideas:
- List three things you're grateful for—past, present, and future.
- Draw an image of something you like—coffee mug, flowers, etc.
- Write down your favorite song lyrics, movie lines, or funny stories.

Try theme days:
- Motivation Monday—Today, I'm going to accomplish…
- Truthful Tuesday—The yucky feelings I'm having today are…
- Wellness Wednesday—The healthy choice I made today was…
- Turtle Thursday—I slowed down to appreciate…
- Faithful Friday—I have faith in my ability to…
- Self-talk Saturday—My affirmation for today is…
- Sacred Sunday—The miracle I noticed today was…

Gratitude Treasure Hunt

Materials: Pen, notebook, radio, five stones, camera, art materials, envelope, stamp, and ingredients to make a healthy beverage.

Instructions: This is a fun game with an important purpose: we're on the lookout for the experience of gratitude. If you want, ask a friend or family member to join you.

1. Make a gratitude list using every letter of the alphabet. I am grateful for: airplanes, bananas, creativity, dreams, energy…

2. Turn on the radio. When the next song starts, dance like no one's watching.

3. Build a cairn with five stones of varying sizes. A cairn is made by placing one stone on top of another. Hikers use them as trail markers. They represent balance and good luck.

4. What's your favorite affirmation? See a list of them in Part IV. Make an affirmation card to place on your dresser.

5. Take seven photos. Find something: old, new, red, blue, beautiful, broken, and blooming.

6. Choose two different people. Leave a note that says, "You're awesome." Mail a card that says, "I'm grateful for you."

7. Buy a book with the word "gratitude" in the title.

8. Write a haiku about peace, love, or nature. A haiku is a Japanese style poem with three lines. The first and third lines have five syllables; the second line has seven syllables.

9. Go to the mirror and say to yourself: "I am beautiful. I am amazing. I am loved."

10. Make a green juice, fruit smoothie, chamomile tea, or hot chocolate. Watch the sunset with someone you love.

PART IV

AFFIRMATIONS

Introduction

During my recovery, a friend of mine, Will, invited me to join his affirmation group. I felt like I'd been thrown a life raft. The purpose of the small group was to send original affirmations through email. I've always liked inspirational things, so I hopped on board.

At first, mine sounded like depressing journal entries, and I wondered if I'd ever send something positive like they did. Eventually, I figured out how to write affirmations, and I discovered the power of positive thinking.

We need to be careful with affirmations. The idea isn't to put on rose-colored glasses to disguise the gray. The object is to gain control of our thoughts and bring them to a higher frequency. It's important that I shared my struggle, rather than skipping over it. We have to start where we are; otherwise, we're just fooling ourselves.

Will told me there's grieving that moves you out of your grief, and there's grieving that keeps you stuck in your grief. Are we getting better or staying sick? Is my grief normal or becoming unhealthy? Once we realize our thoughts create our reality, we begin to take responsibility for our mental chatter.

When I started paying attention to my internal monologue, I was shocked by the harsh words and frequent complaining. When I began to say nice things to myself, it felt odd rather than natural. I had spent so many years beating myself up and undermining my confidence, that it took another year before the affirmations felt believable. The support from the group members gave me strength; it still does.

For a person like me who has a strong inner critic and is prone to self-sabotage, affirmations are a blessing. When I stop practicing them, the dark clouds return and my forward momentum ceases. My inner critic tells me that I'm going to mess up, I don't deserve to be happy, I'm not good enough, and everything I do is wrong. My self-saboteur makes sure I mess everything up to prove my inner critic right. Luckily, my affirmation practice helps me counteract their negative voices. If we believed in ourselves half as much as we doubted, just think of all the things we could do.

The problem is, we easily digest criticism and deflect compliments. We take insults to heart where they erode our self-esteem. We give ourselves permission to be optimistic, especially if this wasn't the norm growing up. We can be healthier than the people around us. Peer pressure is never a good reason to do the wrong thing.

Technically, affirmations need to be written in the present tense, be positive, personal, and specific. It's important to feel the energy behind the words rather than just repeating them like a boring exercise. Over time, you'll begin to embody the positive qualities and making good decisions will be easy. When you believe it, you'll see it, and not the other way around.

Having an affirmation practice gave me the power to throw out the negative tapes and play some refreshing dance mixes. You mean, I don't have to hide my beauty, squander my talents, and dim my light? What a relief! I can challenge my fears and self-doubt. I can soothe my inner child who fears rejection and abandonment. I can make decisions from a place of strength rather than weakness. And this feels wonderful.

Creating a healthy lifestyle doesn't happen overnight, and I still fall off the self-care wagon. I get up, dust myself off, check my pride, climb back on, and get refocused. Making mistakes is how we learn and grow. The wobbly stepping stones teach us more than the sturdy ones. Life is about taking the next step, keeping our balance, and focusing on a successful outcome.

The only way love will come into our lives and feel safe enough to stay, is if we are willing to be honest and vulnerable. The relationships that didn't work out were merely preparation for the ones that will. Being single for the last five years has taught me a lot about *who I am* and *what I want* in a partner. Now, I don't feel anxious or desperate to have someone like me, because I like myself just fine.

Moving out of a deeply entrenched pattern of negative self-talk to begin a practice of positive self-talk is a difficult jump, and the body will have trouble getting there. It's like shifting gears in your car. You don't all of sudden shift to the highest gear. Think of the sun—it rises in the east and sets in the west by making a slow journey across the sky. The process is like walking up a ladder or moving your fingers down the keys of a piano. You didn't get that depressed and down on yourself in one day. It will take some time and effort to improve your mood and self-esteem. Enjoy the ride!

Here's an example of shifting from negative to positive thoughts. "I hate myself. I don't like myself right now. I'm mad at myself. If I weren't such a stupid idiot. Curse words. Okay, that's enough. Take a deep breath. I am confident and capable. I am healthy and strong. Everything's going to be okay. Life is a learning experience. The past is over, and I am free. I have good qualities. My friends like me. God likes me. I like myself. See, this is easy. I am witty and unique. I am a beautiful woman. I love myself."

We work on improving our self-esteem, not to become narcissists with over-inflated egos, so that we can have the life we deserve. Everyone has a special purpose. Everyone has magic inside of them. Everyone gets confused and lonely. No one has it all figured out. No one knows what is best for you. Remember, life isn't a competition. We need to lift each other up. We need space to grow and bloom. We share our joyful experiences to inspire and motivate others. We make a conscious choice to go in the direction of what feels good—deep down soul fulfillment good.

My road to positive thinking hasn't been all sunshine and rainbows. One afternoon, my mom and I were picking our daily affirmation card from Louise Hay's Wisdom Cards. Starting this practice was my idea, and it had been going pretty well. When it was my turn, I shuffled the cards, chose one, and read it aloud. The card must've brought up something, because I got upset and threw some of the cards into the sink that was filled with dishes and soapy water. I dumped the rest of them into the trashcan.

I felt so far away from where I wanted to be. The life-affirming cards threatened my anger and self-hatred, the parts of me that feared change. It's no wonder I became a vibrational match for illness; my emotional energy was of the lowest frequency. A few days later, I bought a new deck, and we started the practice again. This time I was ready to do the work, and I still have the deck!

Here are the affirmations I wrote and sent to my group. Many of them have been edited for length or to make them more general. I have included some of the ones that sound like journal entries, because they are powerful. Most of them are technically correct affirmations, so you can benefit from repeating them. They are organized by theme for easy reference: healing, self-esteem, courage, and faith. I hope you'll feel inspired to start your own affirmation group.

Affirmations for Healing

I am patient with my progress. I can bounce back from this. I have courage to face the day. I have faith in my ability to recover. I am strong and resilient.

∼

I am good enough. I am loved beyond comprehension. I greet the day with gratitude in my heart and a smile on my face. I am learning how to treat myself with loving kindness.

∼

In the moments when I'm ready to give up, I remember there is a deep reservoir of strength within me. When I'm feeling afraid, I remember that it's safe to be me.

∼

I will get out of bed today. My life is waiting for me. I focus on my self-care routine. My environment is peaceful and quiet. I give myself permission to have a relaxing day.

∼

I visualize healing energy circulating through my body. I breathe in, all is well. I breathe out, all is well. I practice compassion and forgiveness. I radiate joy and harmony.

∼

I am a smart, beautiful woman. I make healthy choices. I wear soft, comfortable clothes. I have a job that makes good use of my talents. I am filled with hope and happiness.

I get back into shape by exercising. My heart grows stronger. My body supports me. I am making steady progress. The pain and fatigue are a distant memory.

I take a step back and breathe. My ego wants to go-go-go. My soul is already fulfilled. Today, I will quiet my mental chatter and throw out physical clutter.

My dreams are coming true. The angels are cheering me on. I am excited about my future; it will be a mixture of bold adventure and tranquil reflection.

I remember the past so that I am humbled today. I walked the labyrinth and faced my fears. I am no longer powerless because the truth sets me free. My message is important.

I choose to eat healthy and exercise often. My cells are filled with love and light. I speak my truth in a kind, thoughtful way. I am understood and respected. All is good.

I allow my creativity to flourish. I allow my body to be nourished. I allow people to love me. I give myself credit for my accomplishments. I did a great job!

༄

If this is my highest level of functioning, I accept that. I see myself becoming even stronger than before. I'm going to exercise like I'm on a mission. I deal with reality whether I like it or not. I cry about my losses and then get back into the game.

༄

I am doing the best I can. My best is always good enough. I've been through a lot, even more than I realize. I am a proud survivor. I'll never be the same again, and that's okay. This is a low point in my life. I am learning about resiliency, the strength of my spirit.

༄

Today is my opportunity to feel better, love more, and shine brighter. I can work hard and be productive. I can reach out and make friends. I can relax and have fun.

༄

I can do this. This is easy for me. I am doing great. I have confidence in my abilities. I trust my intuition to guide me. My life will improve when I am nicer to myself.

༄

I remember to loosen up, live a little, all things in moderation. Life is a privilege not a burden. I am ready for my next adventure. I am loveable, tender, and passionate.

༄

Healing energy flows through my body awakening my potential. I forgive others and release the past. I am free to create the life I want. Happiness begins with me.

※

I keep going even when the days are exactly the same. I keep going because I experience breakthroughs. I keep going because the rainbow appears after the storm.

※

I'm not waiting for the day when I feel better. I take the "feeling bad" with me and work it out. I set realistic goals. I do more each day. I make progress. I accept that my life has changed. I find my sense of humor. I laugh out loud, because life shouldn't be this hard.

Affirmations For Self-Esteem

My name is _____ and I love myself.

༒

I am beautiful. I am amazing. I am loved. I choose to sparkle and glow.
I am worthy. I am optimistic. I am confident. I choose to dance and play.

༒

I nurture my inner child with comforting words: "I am here for you. It's going to be okay. I believe in you. I will keep you safe and warm. I am proud of you. You did a great job."

༒

I let the anxiety melt away like ice on a hot day.
I let the fear blow away like leaves on a windy day.
I let the self-doubt hop away like frogs into a pond.
I let the anger burn away like newspapers in a campfire.

༒

I am a creative person, deep thinker, and kind soul. I release my insecurities. The right person will be attracted to me. My personality and character add to my beauty.

༒

I am graceful like a ballerina. I am tough like a football player. I am the sensitive dreamer. I am the loud cheerleader. I always celebrate my uniqueness.

༒

When I breathe, the universe breathes. When I relax, the universe relaxes. I am grounded and centered. My actions are in alignment with my highest good.

∽

I sit in quiet meditation. I focus on my breath. I am filled with love, light, and laughter. Healing begins with me.

∽

I am a productive member of my community. I am a positive role model who makes a difference. The people I meet along the way provide me with information and support.

∽

I have turned the corner and flipped the script. Everything looks the way I imagined it. My life makes sense to me. I am one with the magic. My spirit guides walk with me.

∽

I begin the day with gratitude. I set my intention to have an awesome day. I make it so. It's easy for me to receive and believe compliments. I am a bright and creative person.

∽

I relax and trust. I breathe and release. I journey inward to find my purpose. I follow my heart and live my dreams. I trust my intuition and shine my light.

∽

I am unique like a snowflake. I am brilliant like a raindrop. I am wiser than my fear. I am stronger than my doubt. I am incredibly confident, and my stride becomes a saunter.

∽

I am a warrior of the light. My backpack is filled with scribbled-down notes. I know the way back; I left trail markers. I have so much to share, so much love to give.

∽

I am spiritually driven, emotionally secure, mentally strong, and physically capable. I am planting seeds for tomorrow. I am ready and well prepared. I bloom like a rare flower.

∽

I look out at the purple and orange sunset. The clouds have formed a butterfly, the symbol of transformation; a great sign for today. I have compassion for the new me.

∽

Life is a scared dance. Sometimes, I remember the lyrics but forget the steps. I stumble about messing up the sequence. What's important is that I keep trying. It takes hard work to create a masterpiece. The blood, sweat, and tears are part of the process.

∽

I am a compassionate listener who has strong boundaries. I am treated with respect. My friends enjoy my company. I add depth, meaning, and silliness to our conversations.

∽

Every inch of me is perfect. Every thought is profound. Every action is sacred. Every day divinely led.

∽

I drop into being and focus on my breath. I am pure awareness. I am safe in this moment. I am slowing down to accomplish more. I am witnessing my thoughts as a kind observer. My ego wants everyone to like me. My soul already knows I am divine.

Affirmations for Courage

When I look back, my failures made me stronger. My victories gave me hope. My scars remind me of where I have been. I am a warrior in pink. I bless everything that needs my love. I can rewrite the script, play a better part, go out on a limb, and make a new start.

∽

I am courageous like a samurai warrior. I am disciplined and focused. I move through space with energy and grace. I move through time with a peaceful mind.

∽

My creative work is important. I hear the whispers of my soul calling. Dare I answer? Yes, I must embark on my mission, fearlessly continuing despite the mountains that look so steep. And when I realize the mountains are merely a mirage, I laugh out loud.

∽

I am my own best friend. I am always here for me. My life is improving in the best possible way. My choices reflect the love I have for myself and others.

∽

When I pursue my passions, I walk through the fire untouched. When I am grateful, everything I have is enough. When I love myself, everything I do is enough.

∽

It's important to take breaks when I need to rest. The answers come to me when I have stepped away. There's always enough time to get the important things done.

※

I find open space where I can think clearly. I reconnect with nature. I reaffirm my commitment to being healthy. This is my sacred time and relief. I am blessed.

※

I have the lion's courage, hawk's grace, and turtle's speed. I can blend in like a chameleon, walk tall like a giraffe, or clown around like a monkey. I can run fast like a cheetah, or I can just be me.

※

As I follow my passions, the Universe provides for me. As I process my feelings, I am healing my heart. The bridges I build lead me to exciting places. The doors I take lead me to magical places. I am safe here. I am loved here. I am known here.

※

I am jazzy, simply fantastic. My soul speaks of joyful possibilities. I've always had the map; I just chose to be lost. I've always had the strength; I chose to be weak. I've always been brave; I chose to be afraid. I am ready to begin my spiritual journey.

※

My sensitivity is a gift. I protect my heart because it's easily bruised. I stand up to the bullies, and they quickly back down. They want to shine their light like me, but they are afraid. They are hurting, and so they want to hurt me. It's important to remember this.

I choose the path with heart. My soul dances in delight. Ladybugs gather, four-leaf clovers appear, and dragonflies shimmer. I watch nature's theatrical performance surrounded by my angels. We are the courageous ones, we are the lucky ones.

I am optimistic about my future. I am confident and capable. I am healthy and strong. Success brings me the freedom to travel and explore the world.

I am the artistic muse. I am the wise mystic. I am the seductive temptress. I am the enchanted queen. I am the naïve princess. I am the powerful goddess.

I have pep in my step, a smile on my face, and joy radiating from my heart. I make good decisions regarding my career path. I am worthy of this great opportunity.

Love is my frequency. I love myself to the core. Peace is my reality. I have perfect health. My angels are always near me. I am cherished and adored.

I am tough, becoming tougher, the toughest version of myself.
I am wise, becoming wiser, the wisest version of myself.
I am brave, becoming braver, the bravest version of myself.

I am happy when I march to the beat of my own drum. I am divinely feminine; this is my strength and power. I am healing. I am healer. I am healed.

∽

I am here in the future I imagined in the past. My dreams have become reality. I feel the amazing potential in each moment. I reach out and grab the good stuff. This is fun!

∽

I am grateful for my friends who push me to up my game. I discover my passion—the thing that makes me light up, come alive, and shake off the dust. I have so much to offer the world. I whisper sweet compliments in my ear. I am the coolest of the cool.

Affirmations For Faith

I believe in miracles. My angels dance with me. We have a roaring good time. Happiness comes from being loved. I am grateful for my many blessings. God is good.

෴

I have faith in God's timing. My soul chose this body to learn these lessons. I listen to beautiful, soothing music. Amazing things are possible when I let my soul shine.

෴

I turn toward the light like a flower toward the sun, so that I might see my blessings and be nourished by them. I ask the light to renew my hope and strengthen my faith.

෴

Dear Cupid, please heal the wounded souls everywhere today, especially mine. Show me how to be calm in the face of love. Show me how to be daring and vulnerable. Amen.

෴

I honor my soul purpose. I know what is true for me. The Universe clears a path for me. The real work feels divine and magical. I pray for guidance and protection.

෴

God, give me the strength to remain steadfast. Give me the courage to complete my projects instead of starting new ones. Show me how I can be of service. Amen.

∽

I imagine best-case scenarios. I channel my inner wisdom. I calm my hurried brush strokes. I relax my tense muscles. It is easy for me to be spontaneous and carefree.

∽

I can awaken, enlighten, inspire, motivate, and educate. These are the duties of a warrior. So be it. I reach for the cure, I am the cure. I search for the truth, I am the truth.

∽

I hold your dream in my heart where I keep it safe and protected. I live my dream every day. My relationships are sacred and loving. We are constantly learning and evolving.

∽

I am warm, safe, loved, and understood. I am exactly where I should be. Life is good. When I shine my light and share my truth, I am an inspiration to others.

∽

Dear Goddess, give me an adventurous spirit so that my fairy tale comes true. Give me the whimsy to get carried away. Give me the clarity to see through the haze. Amen.

∽

I look at my to-do list with patient eyes. Instead of feeling overwhelmed and depressed, I feel gratitude for each item. I do one thing at a time. I am a master at getting things done. I am ahead of schedule. I have already crossed the finish line.

∽

I choose peace of mind, breathing deeply. I have peace of mind, breathing deeply. My soul is smiling. My faith is strong. My love is deep. My joy is blooming.

∽

I am a student here to learn. I never claimed to have all the answers. I must remember these lessons are for my own good. It's always darkest before the dawn.

∽

My angels give me hope when I'm feeling down. They hold the pain when it gets too heavy. In my darkest hours, I have seen the light. They tell me there's always more love.

∽

I am magnificent. I am the singer of psalms. I am the collector of wisdom. I am the trash on the curb. I am the mud in the puddle. I am the breath in my chest.

∽

I choose forgiveness over resentment. I choose creativity over stagnation. I choose discipline over laziness. I choose organization over disharmony.

∽

Love makes me sit up straight and think twice about slouching. Love pushes me out of bed and into the shower. Love cheers me up when I'm feeling down. Love gives me strength. Love gives me wings. Love gives me courage. Love gives me all things.

∾

My recovery is now complete. My heart is pure and my mind is clear. Love is my reward. Love is my prize. The Universe aligned our paths without blinking an eye.

∾

Dear Goddess, help me to live another day with gratitude in my heart. I pray for your protection as I begin this new journey. Make me a seeker of truth, believer of love, and warrior of peace. Keep me in your sight and remind me to be brave. Amen.

PART V

POETRY

Introduction

During my recovery, writing poetry helped me to process my experience. I couldn't think of good titles, so I named them colors. What's important is that I was able to express my desires and frustrations. I felt comfortable writing poetry because I didn't think there were many rules, and if there were, I heard the coolest poets always broke them. Do you like to write poetry? I have a feeling it could help you, too.

RED

I get so tired of living like this.
Which version of the story should I bother with tonight?
I'll go with the one that makes us feel all right.
I want you to hold me when I'm falling apart.
I need you to help me make a new start.
I keep waiting for things to get better and they keep getting worse.
This cancer has forced me to focus on myself,
the person I was running away from.
Just leave me alone there's no reason to act like you don't know.
I told you from the beginning, I'm the one fighting.
And you couldn't just be my man.
Better for me, I've learned how not to need.
You were watching me watching you. I was waiting for our love to bloom.
I remember the look of sadness you had for me. I never wanted your pity.
I wanted your love. I've always been strong, now I'm sicker than a dog.
I still can't believe it happened.
I should've gone to a psychic, so she could've pulled the death card.
I used to be excited about my future, now it's just another day.
I never asked for this, not out loud, not outright.
I spend my days wondering what everyone else is doing.
At night, I dream of death putting needles in my steering wheel.
Maybe this detour is warranted, I have to be here to finish this.
This is my healing room, my sanctuary from the storm.
You're passing through picking up souvenirs.
There's no charge, everything is free.

ORANGE

There are leaves on the trees now just like that. I look out the window and the trees are less barren as if the limbs got lonely and asked for some company. They shiver and shake dancing to a beat I wouldn't know. I don't dance anymore. Maybe they're speaking to me, but I haven't been listening. They know what it's like to be stuck in the mud, in between faith and faithless, giving up and going on. I haven't spoken to anyone all day. At night, something'll tickle my funny bone and laughter will clear away my gloom. It's the best part of my day, gets the cobwebs out of my brain.

How could you love me when I don't love myself? I'm sick of everything. I'm sick of this mess. I've got to stay strong and carry on—for me this time. I pray that I can give myself a whole day off from this nonsense. I pray for a love that makes the days less hard. I pray for a love that heals every, "You are wrong." Tell me how to get there, I need directions. Tell me we can watch the game together, I want to relive my glory days.

I remember when everything was perfect, the calm before the storm. I had a sense of impending doom. The cancer was working on me. My guardian angel was trying to warn me. I'm an idiot for talking instead of listening. I'll find my way out of this. I always do. I want my life to be an amazing adventure. All I have are my memories of the good old days. Give me one reason to love you, and I'll leave this sadness behind.

YELLOW

I run from the bad guys, I have no choice.
They're laughing at me. They know something I don't know.
They can see my future in the blink of an eye.
Don't I get some kind of warning?
Spider in the hallway, lights flickering.
I've learned to pray regardless, because even the good days scare me.
Fingers crossed—knock on wood—four leaf clover—rainbow.
I believe this is going to save me; this passion I know won't slay me.
I hang onto myself, the only thing I have left.
Nobody understands why I don't come around.
I've created so many rules I can barely move.
Why did this happen to me?
I can blame it on my genes or simply bad luck.
I can blame it on the water or the rising cost of oil.
Just don't blame it all on me, I beat myself up enough.
I've lost everything that I loved. My heart is broken.
I'll put the pieces back together better than before.
Perform alchemy on my negative thoughts.
Death is easy; it's living that's hard.
I miss your arms around me. I miss being involved. I miss it all.

GREEN

Love, lies, apple pies, you have the most amazing eyes.
I'm slowly going crazy because I don't trust myself.
I've let them get under my skin, now I'm sinking to swim.
I want to take a break, have some tea and cookies.
I went to the grocery and parked the car just once.
Good day for me.
I saw you there and you saw me.
I wonder what you think, is it just curiosity?
It was a busy Friday. The parking lot was full.
Everybody was grabbing food from the shelves.
Preparing for the snow we're supposedly getting.
I keep making the same mistakes.
Am I ever going to grab the bull by the horns?
Wrestle him to the ground and kiss him on the cheek.
Tell him that he's met his match.
This is going to be a good one.
Knock your socks off, make you love me.
I listen for you to knock on my door.
All I hear is the sound of silence.
I can't cook to save my life, thank god for the microwave.
Why did the bagger put a can of soup in with the bananas?
Now they're bruised and broken just like I am.

BLUE

Someday I will let someone trace the tracks of my tears. Maybe in time I can forget when the dementia sets in and the wind rattles my bones. I will let the birds build a nest in the space above my neck. I used to be smart now I think through the fog. I can't hear you. What went wrong?

You've found someone else, she looks like the old me, long hair and pretty. Seeing the two of you together almost brought me to my knees. I managed to stay upright and act like nothing was wrong. I remembered to breathe and smile. You knew the truth when you caught my eye. I pretend to be happy for you. I pretend she's the one for you while I sit here waiting until my last chance is gone. I'm an idiot for harboring these unrequited feelings. I'm in love with longing.

I've forgotten how it feels to be happy. I've been dead so long. Tell them to stop pushing food under the door, this isn't a Kafka novel. Tell them the medication doesn't work, this isn't an insane asylum. Help me to be calm. Help me to stay strong. Tell me to come out of hiding. Tell me the nightmare is over. I won't be a know-it-all hippie chick. I won't be mean. I will enjoy the tiniest gesture. I will enjoy my life forever.

BROWN

You have hungry ghosts in your closet; they eat the life out of all your jokes. They wake you in the night scrambling your sheets, dropping spiders in your mouth while you turn over and pray for morning. The ghosts are mourning your losses because you get what you deserve. You didn't protect me. You stood there smiling and telling me lies. Now, the look of horror still lingers in my eyes. I'm supposed to be grateful because it wasn't that bad. Try walking in my shoes before you say another word.

I'm somewhere else, the master at dissociation. How much pain can one body take? You'll never understand. I took the treatment to live, but this isn't living. If this is living, I'd rather be dead. I'd better be careful with my words, for you'll take me seriously and use my words against me. I can't erase the tracks of my tears. I'm the big cat who devours its kill. I'm the walking dead oblivious to a normal feeling. These scars reveal too much. I'm past the point of rescue. I can't stand the sight of you.

I don't have any privacy because you never stop monitoring me. Cancer is a stigma, a scarlet letter, a curse. You want this to be over—wrapped neatly with a bow. Everything back to normal would take a miracle. I can agree with you that red is blue. I can rig the odds in your favor, uncork the bubbly, and celebrate your victory. I can make you happy at my expense. I can make myself miserable. I can make myself disappear. But I won't.

PURPLE

I can't compete with the pretty girls.
They are experts at makeup and shoes.
I spend my time staring at the moon.
I think your intelligence is sexy.
I think your kindness is beautiful.
I want to hear you say that I'm alive.
Tell me I'm not a disappointment in your eyes.
I can buy my own pickles, but I can't open the jar.
I sit here eating dinner alone, and everything stays the same.
I'm wearing my yellow Life Is Good shirt.
Help me believe in all the things I preach about.
I've become what I loved. I've become you in a way.
I'm going to let your loving hands ease my pain.
It's been five years and it hasn't gone away.
I don't have to put on a show for you.
Maybe a few tricks to keep it interesting.
You see the real me, my essence, my spirit.
The courage you give me is priceless.
Every day, you've been cheering me on.
But you're just another man who feels sorry for me.
I do enough of that already.
I have work to do, and I need to do it alone.
I don't have time to make your life bloom.

PINK

I cry on Wednesdays because you used to be here.
I used to be here before I became a ghost of myself.
I cry on Wednesdays because the pain doesn't go away.
It's my never-ending story and you're tired of hearing about it.
Before I became a ghost of myself, I made a difference in the world.
They wonder why I've stopped talking.
I don't have words for what's happened.
You can draw your own conclusions.

I cry on Wednesdays. Wouldn't you?
It doesn't change anything. How could it? Why would it?
I cry on Wednesdays; it seems like the thing to do.
"You're beating a dead horse. Get over it."
I am the dead horse. Nothing changed in your happy little world.
Your heart still goes beat—beat—beat like it should.
You don't get exhausted before noon.
You don't hate everything that moves.

These could be the good days. What if they are?
What if this is my highest level of functioning?
What if the damage can't be undone?
I had better start living out loud so everyone can hear me.
Or at least quiet as a mouse so the mice can hear me.
I'm not answering the phone; I have too much to say.
I have nothing to offer, nothing you want.
I hope you meet someone you don't have to figure out.
I hope you meet someone who doesn't cry on Wednesdays.

GRAY

Tell me how to make sense of the nonsense. *The way out is through.*
Tell me you'll remove the broken glass. *Your tears have an off-switch.*
Tell me to have compassion for my flaws. *We're going camping.*
Tell me to believe in myself. *Focus on your dreams.*
Tell me to cry tears of relief. *The nightmare is over.*
Tell me the bitterness goes away. *Practice the art of forgiveness.*
Tell me to stop running from my feelings. *You're wasting your good days.*
Tell me the truth. *You have to work twice as hard.*

Tell me why we stare at the television all day. *Entertainment.*
You were made to love me. I've always been the one. *You are one of many.*
Tell me something. Silence is a crummy answer. *Silence is the truth.*
You never know what I'm thinking. *You think too much.*
I don't know how to have a good time. I'm too uptight. *Relax child.*
Tell me to get a life and leave you the hell alone. *The world needs you.*
Tell me that you love me. *Everything is all right.*
Tell me to be grateful. *Think of your highest good.*

I'm wasting my time. I have nothing to say. *Don't go there.*
Tell me to believe in this; it's all I have. *Trust me for once.*
This time, I'm running towards something. *Towards much needed relief.*
Our words fail us every time. *Don't use words.*
I can find the words when I make art. *Buy some markers and paper.*
I'm scared to leave the house. *Nothing bad is going to happen.*
If I really want to do something, I'll find a way. *I believe in you.*
Tell me why everything looks different. *You have perspective.*

Tell me I'm going to finish the book. *Spirit decides when things are done.*
What I wouldn't give for a fruit smoothie. *They aren't that hard to make.*
I don't have any patience. *You have more than you did.*

The treatment saved me, I'm not dying now. *Everything is always dying.*
Tell me to smile instead of this frown. *Wake up and smell the coffee.*
Tell me who I am because I forget. *Remember your divinity.*
Tell me to go to hell. *They have no use for you there.*
Tell me love isn't a game to him. *It isn't a game to him.*
Tell me someday soon. *Someday soon.*

GOLD

I try to be everything to everyone.
I end up being nothing to no one.
I'm chasing something that can't be caught.
I'm out of breath, dripping in sweat.
I convince myself this is enough.
He doesn't know anything about me.
I'm going to catch the next train out of here.
Fear is the only thing standing in my way.
My life is filled with gossip and glitter.
You're the only one who gets the joke.
Sometimes I pretend we're still together.
You're in the kitchen making something for dinner.
Peter Murphy is playing on the stereo.
We had a good life together.
You could've helped me with this, everything—all of it.
We had our chance and time goes so fast.
It takes losing everything to learn the value of things.
I didn't love myself; therefore, I couldn't love you.
Maybe there's a coffee on the counter for you.
And nobody does anything they don't want to do.
I'm waiting for the circus to come to town.
I've practiced being a silly acrobat for you.
We can catch a falling star together.
Dance until dawn with our sneakers on.
While the campfire burns our mistakes.

SILVER

Have a little faith. I'm as tough as nails.
I've found my voice even though I can't hear.
You tell me you love me, but you're not the one.
You don't get to be worried. You cause as much sorrow.
I'm light years ahead of you, and you punish me for this.
Cancer is a tough lesson. I thought this would change you.
It is. It has. Nothing is ever good enough. I'm never good enough.
My muscles are clenched so tightly my entire body is in a knot.
The girl with ten pairs of jeans wears sweatpants.
Guys turn away. I'm an alien, a weirdo.
I've gotten used to it. My ego is on an extended vacation.
Some people look good; it's just what they do.
We don't always choose healthy ways to cope with our traumas.
Stop! You're no problem at all.
I listen to my inner voice—not what others want me to do.
You have to fight and fight and then keep fighting.
Find a glimmer of hope, even if it's a fantasy.
Just don't get run over chasing your dreams.
Look both ways and knock before you enter.
You know the password and the secret handshake.
Make peace with the fact that he'll never be yours.
Find someone who can put air in your tires.
And never tires of your smile.

AQUA

I'm the strongest person I know.
The day we're going to die is tattooed on our heart.
I've lost two pounds of tears remembering how I've spent these years.
Give me a rousing applause or a frown of disapproval.
At this point, I don't trust either of them.
I'm tired of people telling me who I should be.
Did God make us all the same?
Days turn into nights, and I watch the pink sunset alone.
Am I doing the right thing or wasting my youth?
Are these synchronicities enough to keep going?
I'm getting old. I smell defeat. It smells worse than stinky feet.
I'm running out of hope. I'm running on fumes.
I'm forcing my frown into a smile which is worse than a frown.
I want to treat my body like a temple instead of a garbage disposal.
I've been pushed to the side of the road where I can go at my own pace.
Reaching the finish line seems damn near impossible.
I'm the one to blame. Write down my name.
Sign my name! I've forgotten it anyway.
I'm holding onto regret and pinching pennies.
Just marry her, so I can really be sorry.

MAGENTA

I won't let gravity win. Get over here and pick me up.
Help me fight back, give me a will to live.
I smell popcorn burning. Tell me you're not with her.
I won't let this sickness win. The ants move faster than I do.
This is all in my mind.
I'm counting up the reasons why you don't like me.
Because you'll never, ever understand.
We forget the dead and move on.
We find replacements and drink the night away.
I had another bad dream.
Death strangled a man in the hallway.
I didn't say a word. I knew it was going to happen.
I went to pick up some papers on the floor.
He told me, "Those aren't yours."
He was wearing a baseball cap this time.
He got it from his last victim. He was trying to be incognito.
I haven't seen him in awhile, and his return scared me.
It's like he was saying, "Look what I can do."
We were in an employee break room.
The man got something out of his locker and left the room.
Those were his final moments.
He didn't get to say "goodbye" or "I love you" one last time.

PART VI

MY SPIRITUAL JOURNEY

CHAPTER ONE

Meeting Sunny

My spirit guide came to me when I was in a very dark place and gave me the courage to continue. Another day of pain and misery stretched out before me like a road going nowhere. I was in the bathroom getting ready to brush my teeth. I looked in the mirror and said to myself, "I don't know how much more of this I can take."

All of a sudden, I heard a male voice say, "Hey, Tiger Girl! What are you doing out here in the forest up in a tree?"

I definitely heard him, but I asked, "What did you say?"

He repeated himself, which made me happy.

My mom was downstairs in the kitchen, and I knew she didn't hear him. My initial reaction to meeting him was hesitation. I don't like spooky things. Everybody wants something. How am I going to explain this? I'm not. I'll keep it secret. I had enough to deal with getting through the day. My family already thought I was different, and I wasn't ready to add another log to that fire.

I've always believed in angels, but I didn't think I had any. I guess I'd never taken the time to make their acquaintance. It was me who was afraid to accept the gift I'd been given. He came into my life to make things better, not worse. I could say I was being cautious. A better explanation—I excelled at pushing good things away. Luckily, he stayed with me.

I could feel his warm energy and gentle presence standing right next to me. I quickly finished up in the bathroom because I knew the words were coming. I began to hear dialogue and see characters. I went into my bedroom and picked up a yellow tablet of paper sitting on my dresser. My to-do list was on the first page. I flipped to a clean page, grabbed a pen, and wrote a story about a girl who becomes a shaman to heal her sick boyfriend. It was a safe way for me to start processing my cancer experience.

He was giving me something to do until the headaches went away, and I discovered my love for writing. When I moved out of my mom's house into an apartment, I had a feeling I'd be able to talk with him again. Sure enough, my imaginary friend kept me company, balancing my tears with laughter.

Like Neale Donald Walsch's *Conversations with God*, I was at the end of my rope and needed an explanation for why my life derailed. I asked Sunny questions and wrote down his answers, creating a back and forth dialogue. I filled many pages of my notebook, scribbling furiously to get everything written down.

Looking back, this doesn't surprise me. I had stopped talking to almost everyone except my mom, which I don't recommend. There's a reason support is called support; it holds you up, so you don't fall down. My loneliness must've prompted this strange relationship and, ironically, I felt safe talking to him.

He told me rather kindly, "I'm here to help you, and we can help others. Get to work, start writing. Do this or else you'll never be free." I understood what he meant, and I trusted him even when I doubted myself.

At the same time, I was denying myself the comforting perks of a real relationship: shoulder massages, cooking delicious meals, watching movies, and taking fun adventures together. Dating after cancer was an even scarier prospect than talking with a ghost. I felt broken and fragile, like damaged goods moved to the clearance table. At least the thought of chasing emotionally unavailable men no longer appealed to me. My tolerance for drama and heartbreak was gone, and I began to crave real love again.

Sunny was a true friend; he didn't judge me or require perfection. He didn't care if my hair was messy and my clothes were out of style. He could see my tiger spirit was being held captive by my fears and insecurities. He wanted to help me get unstuck.

It's called clairaudience (clear hearing) when you can hear Spirit. And even though talking with angels is common, I worried what people would think. I started second guessing myself again, and stepped away from the manuscript. Finally, I decided it was happening for a reason. Something good would come from this—if nothing else, he helped me. I don't want to let anyone down, especially Sunny.

Our conversations were filled with love and laughter. He depended on me when I felt useless. He believed in me when I had given up hope. I know nothing for sure except certainty is a myth, and when Spirit talks, you listen. Recently, when I was trying to chalk up his existence to mere hallucination, he told me, "Don't act so surprised. You know the veil between life and death is thin and luminous."

My introduction to the Spirit world actually started when I was in college. My boyfriend and I frequented new and used bookstores. Ian helped me pick out books to read, and some of them profoundly affected me. The first one I enjoyed reading was Erica Jong's *Fear of Flying*, and I thought to myself, "Someday I'm going to write a book."

The other was Jane Roberts' channeling book, *Seth Speaks*, which I finished reading even though it scared me. Her book opened my eyes to the idea of energy personalities, multiple dimensions, and prepared me for meeting Sunny.

Before I was born, my soul chose the lessons I'd go through and the helpers I'd need. Sunny is a spirit guide rather than a guardian angel, because he's lived in human form. One way to connect with your spirit guide is through automatic writing.

Automatic writing is the activity of letting words flow freely onto the paper without stopping to edit them. Write whatever comes to mind. Ask specific questions. It takes time and practice. Don't get discouraged. You will find the answers come to you while you're taking a walk, brushing your teeth, or washing the car. Keep pen and paper nearby, so you're always prepared.

There's a lot of universal consciousness we can tap into, and we want to make sure we're inviting high frequency vibrations to the party. It might be helpful to say a prayer for protection, "I invite only loving energy into the room. Guide my thoughts in the direction of my highest good. Show me how I can be of service. Amen."

Meeting my spirit guide was caused by a combination of things. I've always been sensitive and intuitive. I believed it was possible. I was struggling and needed assistance. I didn't have a television, so it was pretty quiet in my apartment. I also began turning the radio off, so that I could hear him better. He helped me get through my cancer experience and grieve my father's death.

I used to lay in bed at night typing our conversations on my phone. The next morning, I'd check to make sure it really happened. I know when he's here, and when he's gone helping someone else. Even though I'm glad to be doing better, I miss him sometimes. Down the road, I might try automatic writing again and see what happens. For now, I'm content with the connection I made and the help I received.

Technically, it's a form of channeling, but my skills are very basic. He doesn't take over my body, nor talk through me. When I'm at my computer, sometimes I can feel him standing next to me. When I picture him, he has an ethereal body; he isn't solid like us. I don't hear him talking out loud, I hear his voice in my head; it isn't audible to other people. I've noticed, if I'm not careful, my ego will rush ahead and answer for him.

I think everyone has psychic abilities and extrasensory perception. For some, it's underdeveloped and takes practice. For others, it feels normal and natural. As kids, we're allowed to use our imagination. When we grow up, we're taught to trust science. Even the greatest geniuses admit there's something beyond science that's unexplainable, magical, and divine.

It takes strength to listen, faith to believe, and courage to share. The dialogue that follows is from our conversations. When I asked for his name, he said, "You can call me your friend." And then I heard the name, "Sonny." I spell it "Sunny" because he became my light in the darkness.

CHAPTER TWO

Message of Hope

How can I love more? It takes so much energy. (Julie)

Love creates more love, and fear creates more fear. (Sunny)

I usually feel either angry or sad.

How's that working for you?

Not good.

Didn't think so.

I'm afraid to talk to you.

You're scared.

I don't know if I can tell people I hear a voice. They might lock me up.

This isn't the first channeling book, and it won't be the last.

Why me?

You're listening. You've suffered a great deal, which has altered your reality. I'm helping you; in turn you'll help others. You have a big heart and lightening sharp perception. Sensitive souls must learn how to protect themselves. It took nearly dying for you to slow down. It took losing everything for you to learn gratitude. Because of all this, you can give a voice to the voiceless.

Good night! You make me sound so cool. I struggle every day with the heavy burdens I place on my shoulders. I'm a control freak who yearns to have fun. I live in this self-imposed exile. My anxiety is going to be my undoing. I've forgotten how to be happy.

Happiness hasn't forgotten you. Life is simple and you make it difficult. You can stop punishing yourself any day now. You didn't do anything wrong.

I've always been hard on myself.

You worry yourself ragged and sabotage your success. You're waiting for permission to pursue your dreams. You're too stubborn to accept the help you need. You're too timid to welcome the love you need.

I feel as though my heart has shrunk. The chemotherapy squeezed it to death and crushed my hopes. I've given up on love.

Love hasn't given up on you.

Love should run for the hills.

You're funny, funnier than you realize. You have so much love to give, but you keep it all to yourself. You've grown stingy.

I'm done giving for now.

You can't turn giving on and off; it isn't a light switch. You act like you don't care, but you do. You wouldn't be writing this if you didn't care.

Why stay here with me in this room? It can't be that exciting.

Because you need company. You were slipping away…

And you saved me, I remember.

Do you remember what I said?

Hey, Tiger Girl! What are you doing out here in the forest up in a tree?

So, what is your answer?

You're using a metaphor. I'm hiding out. I'm a scaredy cat. I'm not living my purpose. I ran away from danger and now I need help getting down.

You're stuck because you won't let anyone help you. You have to reach out.

I did, finally, after you left. I found someone who can help me. At least, I think.

I'm glad to hear that.

I just have to be careful that I don't scare him away.

Take it slow.

I will.

You were caught up in your pain and couldn't find gratitude.

I was in a lot of pain; it's hard to be grateful for pain.

Pain is a teacher.

I'm tired of learning.

Until you understand, the same lesson will haunt you.

What do I need to understand?

You worry about the wrong things. Your "flaws" make you beautiful. Why do you want to be like everyone else?

I just want to be me.

You can be.

I'm trying to keep my feet planted firmly on the ground.

What fun is that?

Guess it's not possible anyway. The other day on my walk this dragonfly wouldn't leave me alone, like it was trying to tell me something.

Maybe it was.

I don't speak dragonfly.

What do you think the dragonfly symbolizes?

They have the courage to fly free. They are funny and beautiful.

When you were in Santa Fe, you went to the shamanic journey with your friend, Jennifer. Her therapist acted as a shaman and led a drum circle so you could discover your animal spirit guides. What did you discover?

Well, the drumming put me to sleep. In my dream state, I entered the tunnel and came through a tiny hole in the creek bank across the street from my mom and dad's house where I grew up. I walked around the dry creek bed, when all of a sudden a white tiger swallowed my arm and then the rest of me. I was looking out from inside the white tiger. I became the white tiger.

You shape-shifted into a white tiger. And then what happened?

A black panther approached me. I could tell he was kind and wouldn't hurt me. I think I even petted him. I understood he would walk beside me as my protector.

Interesting, and yet you're so fearful.

There are things to fear.

You create most of your fears.

My bad.

You have another concern. I can see it on your face.

I'm afraid I'm dying, and now I want to live. What if it's too late?

Why do you think you're dying?

I think I have cancer again, a recurrence. I'm stressed out. I'm not being healthy. I'm letting everyone down. What if I have to go through all that again?

Relax, take a deep breath, and be in the moment. Be good to Julie. Show her the same compassion you show others. Let go of everyone else's expectations. You'll never be able to please them.

I feel better already. I can still hear their nagging voices.

What do they say?

Save me. Help me. How dare you! Who do you think you are? You must suffer like us and fall in line.

Can you help them?

Maybe.

Help yourself first, and then you'll be able to help them. Understood?

Understood. I'm as slow as the seven-year itch. I don't know why they want my help anyway.

They don't want your help. They want to control you. You've gotten faster, almost too fast. You're about to go back to your old ways of running yourself ragged; don't do that.

What are you talking about?

The cancer slowed you down, way down.

The radiation slowed me down to a crawl.

There's nothing wrong with that.

The world moves a bit faster than that.

It doesn't have to. You're choosing the speed.

I guess so.

Spreading a message of hope doesn't require all that much.

I had a frown on my face for most of the day. I'm the least likely candidate for spreading hope. How about sadness? I can spread that 'til the cows come home.

It's hope we need to focus on.

Why?

Because hope gets you out of bed in the morning. Do you remember that article about suicide?

I do.

What is the one thing that saves a person from committing suicide?

Hope.

Yes, having hope that things will get better and their situation will change. There is a huge distance between hope and hopelessness.

I've been on both ends of the spectrum. Hope floats.

You're worthy and deserving of a good life. He didn't choose the bottle over you. He was powerless to alcohol; it's called an addiction for a reason.

I understand that now.

Your inner child is still crying out for attention.

She's a whiny baby. I don't drink much anymore. I miss it sometimes.

Moderation, otherwise it's just a way to numb out.

I know.

I think that's your favorite phrase. If you know so much, then act like it. Cut this helpless-little-girl bit.

I don't act like a helpless little girl.

Sometimes you do.

CHAPTER THREE

Letting Love In

Why do I struggle so much? (Julie)

You struggle because you don't trust yourself. If you could trust yourself, then you might be able to trust someone else. (Sunny)

I doubt it.

You struggle from the moment you get up until the moment you go to bed.

That's what I know.

What would happen if you stopped struggling?

I'd be happier.

And that's way worse than struggling. I'd definitely pick struggling.

Now, you're laughing at me.

You don't have to struggle to prove to the world that you can struggle. "Hey world, I can bear these hard times. I can be a trooper." Show the world you love yourself. "Hey world, I can take care of myself. I can be happy!" That would be a healthy role model.

It would be.

You need daily soothing.

I know that.

If you know so much, then why don't you make some changes?

I'm trying.

You're squeaking by, barely making the effort. You walk around with your sad eyes and worried look. You have all the time in the world to present yourself in a way that's more presentable.

I'm pulled in five different directions.

Not anymore.

I do have a bit more freedom than I used to.

Feels good, doesn't it? With freedom comes responsibility. You have to be your own boss and set your own schedule.

Yes, it does. And yes, I do.

I know whose love you need.

What? Where did that come from? When will I meet him?

When you believe in yourself, you'll believe in him.

I don't have room for love.

That's the only thing you have room for.

I'm not ready.

Precisely, and that's the vibe you put out there, so they turn away confused. What are you so afraid of?

I don't want to be hurt again.

That's funny, coming from the person who usually does the hurting.

Hey, watch it!

You think you can protect yourself from getting hurt, when it's twice as dangerous to go without love. Reaching out takes practice. Take baby steps and test the waters. Small accomplishments strengthen your confidence. There's nothing to be afraid of out there. You don't believe what I know.

What do you know that I don't believe? You've lost me again.

I know that you could make somebody really happy, and they could make you really happy, too.

I had that once.

You think love is a one-time deal, that it has an expiration date? It was a fluke that he loved you? Everybody wants to be loved. Have you ever thought of that?

I struggled today parking my car and going into the store. I got anxious thinking about all the people that would be in there. It's Saturday, not the best day for a quiet outing, and I didn't have much energy to spare.

Well, don't waste it on nonsense. The good thing was—you tackled your fears, pulled yourself together, and bought the stuff you needed.

I looked like a hot mess.

You looked like reality.

Reality is a hot mess?

Yes.

I don't want to cause myself so much trouble. I over-think everything.

You were thinking negative thoughts. You weren't saying your affirmations. You talked yourself out of going into the store. You were watching everyone else.

They weren't struggling. They were happy like I used to be.

You drove around hoping to shake the anxiety, only to find it had gotten worse. Then you started beating yourself up for not being perfect. You kept re-parking the car because you felt unsure of yourself. Your need for the store items finally overcame your fears, and you dragged yourself in there.

I guess you were watching. I make things so difficult. I know better than to do that. Next time, I'll try to enjoy myself.

Just go with the flow.

༄

Is there anything bigger than love? (Julie)

Love is the life force, the beat of the heart, the light in the dark, the spark, and the flame. There's nothing bigger than love, because love is part of everything. (Sunny)

Even hate and fear?

Hate is love that has turned against itself. Everything has potential for good or evil. This duality gives you freedom of choice and creates change. The conditions you know as life wouldn't exist if there weren't also conditions of death. The opposing force has to be in existence.

That's interesting.

You're not missing anything out there.

I'm not?

When you feel better, and you will, you'll be able to return to the world.

It doesn't feel like things are going to get better.

Do you want things to get better?

Yes.

Maybe you haven't rested enough.

I'm tired of resting.

You've been through a lot and expect to bounce back like nothing happened.

I went back to work, and everything was different. I'm no longer that person, and the headaches were excruciating.

It probably worked out for the best; you have a new task now.

I do?

Writing about your cancer experience is helping you get closure.

I've had to fight for the right to write. It takes time and energy. You see a pitcher pitching, a chef cooking; a writer's work is done behind the scenes. Glamorous? Not quite. It's become a labor of love. This is a big project, bigger than I realized.

You could write in a coffee shop.

I could. You're the only one who doesn't want me to be someone else.

I have unconditional love for you.

Thank you. That's the best kind.

You can have true love again.

Sounds groovy.

You'll attract what you are, and right now you're a bit scattered like the leaves in the park. You stumble onto the road feeling unprepared, so you stop for a break. Breaks are fine, but you seem to be on an extended break.

I haven't been feeling good, yet I've been very productive during this time.

You've learned your lesson about speaking up and saying—enough is enough. What works for them doesn't necessarily work for you. Sometimes being with the "in crowd" makes you feel more like an outsider.

It's a ghost town around here.

You need peace and quiet to work.

I need to maintain my sanity. Thank God for music. I need to stop cleaning the apartment and get some writing done. I swear the dust is winning.

Let it win.

I will.

Your illness was a blessing and a curse.

It was hardly a blessing, surely you jest.

Part VI: My Spiritual Journey // 127

I'm afraid not.

My head is heavy from these thoughts.

He loved you, every minute of every day.

Even when he was drinking?

Yes, even then.

That's all he did.

That's not all he did. Sometimes, he was there for you, and you turned away. You need to forgive him. Send him light and love.

I forgive him. I really do.

Don't blame others for your situation. Notice when you're stuck and keep moving. Swim fast and hard. Go around the bend, and see what you haven't seen. Go where you haven't gone. Being under-stimulated isn't good for you.

Why do you put this burden on me?

Your soul purpose will not be a burden to you; it's a gift from God.

I know that now.

You're experiencing no more and no less than you can handle.

I used to beat myself up with my thoughts, now my body is beating me up.

You've experienced a great deal of pain, I won't argue with that. Look at the good that resulted. You've forgiven your dad. You have a better relationship with your mom. You take walks and do yoga. You are writing several books.

I like compliments, keep going!

You have affirmations on your wall that you repeat throughout the day. You want to get better. That being said, it took the lump growing to the size of a marble before you found it. You weren't paying attention to your body.

I took my health for granted. I thought I was healthy. I think most people do. I never dreamed anything bad would happen. Breast cancer didn't even cross my mind. I had a bad feeling about the lump.

You were harboring a fugitive.

He was shooting the place up and stealing the good wine.

It's nice that you can joke about it, shows you're healing.

I cry when I'm alone; it helps.

Your feelings want to be heard and respected. Underneath the hurt is your frustration at not receiving the love you needed.

And how do I receive this love?

First, you have to love yourself. Be perfectly happy alone, so that you don't appear anxious or desperate. When love appears, don't make a big mess of the situation.

Like I did with "Wayne."

Yes. It's okay to push away a sugary substitute that does nothing but make you hungrier for the real thing. Live each day like it's your last. Someday it will be, and you don't want a heart full of regret.

I have that now.

Let it go. Things always work out for the best.

I've been thinking about what happened and trying to make sense of it.

The love of your life is marrying someone else. Now that's nonsense.

You sure know how to cut to the chase. That wasn't what I was talking about, and I don't want to talk about it.

Your old problem. When will you let love in?

No one will ever love me. Not now.

Part VI: My Spiritual Journey // 129

That's not true.

It feels like it.

So you have to rest a bit more than most people. And you have some rituals and phobias. Does that make you unlovable?

No.

Okay then. When someone loves you, they love you despite your faults, not that you have any faults. Smiling again, I see?

Yes. I cracked a smile over your attempt at a compliment.

You need to buy some beer and crack one of them open.

Are you sure you're my spirit guide?

One beer won't hurt. You don't have a drinking problem, and it might take the edge off. It might taste good.

I just wrote "beer" on the store list. I'm looking forward to it. Maybe some pretzels or chips to go along with, now that sounds good.

You don't drink because you like to be in control. You don't mind swimming in your murky emotions, whereas most people don't even want to get their big toe wet.

I think I sacrifice too much for my writing.

You can have whatever you want.

I need some new clothes. I haven't been shopping in awhile.

Clothes are easy to find.

I guess so.

If only you could've let someone help you. You saw sickness as defeat; you put that on yourself. Recovery can be an adventure.

My recovery was a disaster.

If he isn't the one, he'll never be the one. If you want joy, you'll have it. If you want misery, you'll have that.

What if the cancer comes back?

Stop asking, "What if?" It's the quickest way to make yourself go crazy.

I hate myself for what I've become. I've created so many silly rules. I ruin my good days. I'm falling apart. I can't keep it all together. This fight is bigger than me, nothing gets done, and we never get ahead.

You need to get out of your head, connect with people, and have a good time. Relationships help you grow as a person. You spend too much time alone. I'm worried all you're doing is ruminating and nothing gets solved.

What am I trying to solve?

Unsolvable things. Do you think you'll be young and pretty forever?

Who says I'm young and pretty now?

You are when you smile.

Thanks.

You do what's right, and that makes you beautiful. An honest soul is priceless. Don't be afraid of the world. Self-doubt is your downfall.

Easy for you to say.

Do what feels right in your body. Enjoy yourself. Treat yourself like a queen instead of a peasant.

Okay, I'll try.

CHAPTER FOUR

Courage to Fly

You sabotage everything. (Sunny)

I thought that's what I had to do. (Julie)

No, that's what you know how to do.

I'm exhausted before I get started. I'm done. I'm over it.

This isn't you. The Julie I know wouldn't give up.

This is more than I can handle.

God doesn't give you more than you can handle.

It feels like it.

Then feel again.

Everyone else is perfectly fine, and I'm floundering.

What about the guy with the dog?

What about him?

You like him. Have you talked to him?

No. He has a girlfriend and a dog.

I bet he'd be with you, if you got back into the game.

I doubt it.

You don't believe in anything, and that's your problem.

I believe in reality. I believe in my allergies.

Hasn't cancer taught you anything?

Don't wait until my last chance is gone.

What else?

I'm tired of having to be this "changed from the cancer person." What if it changed me for the worse? How's them apples?

Your anger is poison.

Nobody asked you. Leave me to my misery.

You've been negative all day.

I'm down again.

Pick yourself back up. You've done it before, you can do it again.

I've lost my motivation. Everything is wrong.

No. Everything is right; you're just looking at it wrong. You're being pessimistic. The enthusiasm you had yesterday is gone.

I spent the whole day trying to control a situation I couldn't control.

I was watching.

I wondered if you'd be here tonight. Can you read my thoughts?

Yes.

I bet that's weird.

Someday you'll understand. I see where you go astray and how you get stuck. Mistakes help you grow. Life would be very boring if you had it all figured out.

Having it all figured out would be great.

You only think it'd be great. Your need for control has caused your world to become very limited. There are things you want to do, people you want to see, and you fail to reach out. You put so much pressure on yourself to conquer the world. The world doesn't need conquering.

I guess not.

Be grateful for small accomplishments. There will always be something else that needs to be done. You have plenty of time to enjoy yourself along the way.

Doesn't seem like it; seems like I'm under the gun.

You put yourself there.

There's this voice in my head, "How dare you take the day off, how dare you write a book, how dare you…"

Quiet the voice of shame and guilt; it wants you to be unhappy.

Well, I am.

You're a happy person who chooses to be unhappy. You tie yourself up in knots trying to be perfect. Everything is going to be okay. Make your phone calls; get your appointments set up. Otherwise another week goes by.

I don't like to make phone calls and set up appointments.

Put your fears in your back pocket. Pull some courage out of your front pocket and get to work.

I'll probably find more lint than I will courage.

You have more courage than you know.

I have too much to do.

You only think you have too much to do.

Everything is messed up.

Here we go again.

I'm a slow learner.

It's going to take some effort to get back on track.

I'm tired.

Snap out of it, sister. I'm tired of watching you waste away. If you want a better life, you're going to have to work for it.

∽

If this is living, I'd rather be dead. (Julie)

It'll get better, and what doesn't get better, you'll learn to live with. See how much better you're doing than six months ago. (Sunny)

I feel like I've been beaten with a baseball bat.

But you're alive.

Thanks for reminding me. I have chronic pain and fatigue. Every day is a struggle. How can something help me and hurt me at the same time? Isn't that contradictory?

You were fighting fire with fire. Next time choose peace.

Peace isn't one of the treatment options.

Are you sure?

I don't know.

Maybe you could look at your recovery as a challenge.

It bothers me that I used to be perfectly fine. I had it all and it gotten taken from me. No one understands, unless they've been through it.

You had cancer; everything wasn't perfectly fine. Not everything was taken. Some of it you gave away. You look at the past with rose-colored glasses. You're alive now. Doesn't that mean something to you?

I could still have cancer; it could be in remission.

Quite possibly. Cancer is very sneaky. In time, there'll be better treatments that cause less damage. Modern medicine has come along way; it could've been worse.

I doubt it. A part of me died. Good parts of me died. I'm grieving what got taken. I'm grieving what I lost.

What did you lose?

I lost my faith in humanity. I lost my peace of mind. I shook hands with Death, and He laughed in my face. How do I come back to life? I've been somewhere no one should ever go.

BUT YOU ARE ALIVE!

Okay! You don't have to yell; I'm not deaf. I'm done complaining and tired of hearing your answer.

That is the answer.

Doesn't feel like it.

That's because you're bitter. How does that feel?

Not good.

Well?

Well, what?

Choose a new feeling. Forgive the past and let it go. Do your best now.

I have about five minutes of peace between worries. Why do I worry so much?

Worrying makes you feel productive, yet it's counterproductive. It's like rocking in a chair; it gives you something to do, but it gets you nowhere.

I got the short end of the stick when my temperament was chosen.

I can explain more about worrying if you want to listen.

Okay.

What would you rather do than worry?

Be happy, productive, and relaxed.

You can be all those things. You want to plan everything down to the wire. You can't foresee what's going to happen once you leave the house. You used to look forward to new adventures, now you dread them. You've lost your confidence.

How could I let things get this bad?

There's nothing wrong with hitting rock bottom, as long as you don't stay there. You have so much potential, but you squander the moment.

Life is difficult.

You make it difficult.

There's so much pressure on me to get a job. Maybe writing is my job.

Writing is your job right now. Don't feel guilty about following your dreams. Hopefully, you'll let your friends back into your life; they miss you.

I miss them, too. My self-imposed exile is very weird.

You've definitely learned the art of solitude.

What if I'm running from my problems again?

I can't answer that for you.

It won't matter how many books I've written, because I'll still be alone.

Love is worth more than a book deal. He's out there waiting for you to be ready.

You know whose love I need?

I know whose love you need. His love would ease your pain.

I used to chase every guy in town looking for validation.

You chased them while they were running away. You should've chased someone who was running toward you.

Part VI: My Spiritual Journey // 137

I craved drama, and that's what I got.

You gave your power away in order to get it. A man who loves you will want you to keep your power. He'll want you to be strong, so that every once in awhile he can be weak. He can handle your successes and failures. His love will give you strength.

That sounds nice.

You're a strong woman, which is why you have a hard time finding a mate. They know that to be with you will take a tremendous amount of courage and self-reflection. You can demand a great deal because you offer so much. Don't be stingy with your love.

I'm not stingy.

You've become rather stingy.

I'm selective.

You're not selecting anything.

CHAPTER FIVE

Following My Dreams

How will I know when I've found my life's purpose? (Julie)

You'll know without a doubt in every fiber of your being. And yet, even when you feel absolutely certain, you might still choose another path. (Sunny)

Out of fear.

Yes.

I feel happy when I write and a bit scared, which is probably a good thing. It's always like, "Oh my God, am I really going to let myself do what I want to do?"

You don't have to answer to anyone.

I guess not. What if people make fun of our dialogue?

If you believe in this, that's all that matters. I mean no harm and neither do you. You're trying to make sense of the horrible ordeal you went through. People can think what they think.

Okay.

I think you're worrying for nothing. The majority of people believe in angels.

You're right. I'm being the doubter.

Do you remember your dad's painting that was hanging in the family room?

Yes, I do. He painted a picture of a man in a small boat. There's a lighthouse and a larger boat in the distance that he could row toward, but it looks like the dark, murky waters are going to get him.

That's what happens. Don't let it happen to you. You're not your dad. You don't have to go down the same path. He knew what was going to happen. Painting was his art therapy. Those murky waters were his addiction. The small boat couldn't protect him.

He had to leave the large boat.

Addiction took his love and support away. You can have love and support.

Okay.

You don't sound convinced.

I'm convinced.

Our friendship gives you hope, but you're fearful to continue the journey we've begun. You want to work on your safe projects, the stories your ego is writing. Your ego is very conniving. I can only whisper and hope you pay attention.

My ego is pushy and annoying. You are much kinder. Sometimes, I think you're gone, and you're here.

As it should be. You've always known you had something important to write, that one day you'd set off on your own path, quiet their voices, and believe in yourself. You knew how difficult it'd be, which is why you took so many detours. You weren't where you wanted to be, which is why you were so miserable. Your creativity was stifled. Soon, you'll find like-minded people who encourage courage.

I hope so.

I know so.

Must be nice.

I'm not being right in an "I told you so" kind of way. I'm laughing with you and not at you.

Who's laughing?

Oh, your little soul is very happy when we're in conversation.

I am happy, thanks, but why do I feel guilty for following my dreams? I don't have a regular job. My car is the only one in the parking lot. Everyone else is at work.

Feeling guilty is a waste of time, and not everyone is happy to be at work. The Universe is supporting you right now so you can accomplish this task. You feel guilty because you were taught to conform, and you're not conforming. You've had many regular jobs.

I have. You name it, I've worked there. Writing is what I want to do; and yet, I barely give myself enough time to do so.

In time, you'll develop more discipline and give yourself permission.

I let myself get distracted.

Many young people are "doing their own thing" when it comes to employment.

I'm sure that baffles old school parents.

Parents mean well. They want their children to be self-sufficient. Most of the time, it does make sense to choose the safe route because generating cash from creativity can be difficult. That being said, life is about following your dreams. Soul satisfaction feels better than financial security. The trick is to have them both.

A friend and a lover combined.

Exactly.

Picking security over happiness doesn't make sense to me. It's hard to put your heart into work you don't care about. I didn't mind working at the insurance company because I liked my co-workers, and the routine was good for me. It was a job that paid the bills. We were busy and time passed quickly. I worked hard, got promoted to another department, but that made things worse not better.

Now, you'll help people in another way. You have to create your own routine and be productive. You're getting your questions answered. Isn't that what you wanted?

Yes, I just wish I were juicing and eating healthier. I'm a terrible cook.

Cooking isn't that hard.

Well, then you can fix dinner.

Let your soul speak, your heart decide, and your spirit fly.

That sounds nice.

Be brave and listen.

You know more than I do.

It's not about who knows more.

Everything I say you dissect. It sounds like I'm doing everything wrong.

We're using you as an example, and you're taking it personally.

How should I take it?

Take it as trying to reach clarity for everyone. This is about being fearless enough to walk through the fire. Everyone is given a mission.

For many years, I heard the call and turned away.

I was the one calling.

Now, you're being funny.

Laughter is the best medicine.

It is.

What are you so afraid of?

Everything. Success. Failure. Not being loved.

You were happy with Ian. Why don't you let yourself be happy again?

My dad is dead.

That's not a good reason. He wants you to be happy. He died five years ago; your grief has lessened in intensity. He's sorry that he wasn't there for you. He loved you more than you'll ever know. I'm making you cry now. I'll stop.

Sometimes, I think I see him. Do you see him?

Yes, I can see him. This is tearing you up. I'm sorry. The tears come from a well of sadness deep inside your heart.

There's a hole in my heart, that's why the tears are leaking out. I've developed a spiritual relationship with him. He's here on earth, but he can't be with us anymore. He's separated from us. I see him walking on the bike path. I want to scream at him, but I'd be screaming at strangers, and that'd be bad.

Maybe he's here for you now more than he was when he was alive.

That's awful to say.

In some ways it's true.

I think he's still around.

The dead often are.

Sometimes I feel dead inside.

What would make you feel alive?

A boyfriend.

Well, go get yourself one; you've done it before.

Easier said than done. That would require me to be pretty and normal.

Is that so bad?

No. I need to focus on my writing.

It isn't either/or. You can have a boyfriend and writing career, many people do. Don't wait for Prince Charming to knock on your door; he's too busy.

Part VI: My Spiritual Journey // 143

I don't have the energy for a boyfriend.

He'd understand your fatigue.

I doubt it.

He isn't going to ask you to run a six-minute mile, silly.

He might, silly.

You've gotten your physical strength back, for the most part. Now, it's more the mental and emotional stuff.

I realized last night that I've combined my counting and checking rituals with my affirmations. I'm one crazy bird.

If you met someone you liked, don't you think those things would slowly fade away?

Maybe. Probably.

Why do you want to be miserable?

I don't want to be miserable.

Miserable is your new normal. You need to switch gears. Vroom! Vroom!

I'm too busy for a boyfriend. I can't give him what he needs.

They don't need much: support, understanding, love. Listen to your excuses. You're going to excuse yourself out of your due. Love can heal your wounds.

Okay, so I'm afraid. Imagine that, right? It seems to be a common theme for me. I've put myself into a prison of my own making; my life has come to a screeching halt.

There's no magic involved. You just start living again, leave the house, and talk to people. Without people, life is empty and meaningless.

I heard the birds chirping today on my walk, but I had no idea what they were saying. I don't speak their language, either.

Neither do I.

I'd like to be in a relationship someday.

Then someday you will be. Wouldn't that be great?

Very great.

⁂

You put me at the end of the book. They're never going to find me. (Sunny)

Now, who sounds egotistical? Or are you being facetious? (Julie)

You're afraid to share this experience. You're more comfortable with the facts and figures. You're caught up in the story instead of the feelings beneath the story.

Feelings are messy.

You need to aim your arrows in the right direction; otherwise, you'll keep missing the target. Unless you're trying to miss the target on purpose. I hope not.

I go back and forth between hope and hopelessness.

Until you can trust again, I'll be your friend.

Thank you.

We hear more in the silence than we do in the noise. We hear cries for help.

Is that where you are some days, most days?

Yes, I have other people to help.

How come?

People have free will; they make a big mess of their lives and then wonder why they're unhappy.

Like I did.

Like you did.

Glad we agree on something. Do you remember the two dreams I had about Death?

Describe him to me.

He looked like a normal guy, but I knew he was the living dead. His eyes were green and weird. He seemed unusually kind for being Death.

Maybe Death is kind.

I was drawn to his house, even though it had an ominous feeling. The yard was in an upheaval with mounds of dirt. It was nighttime, like in the scary movies. Luckily, there were moon, porch, and street lights. I walked up the driveway, I couldn't turn back. I had to knock on the door and see what was on the other side.

Sounds very cliché, but that's exactly what you were doing. Nobody wants to die, yet everyone is curious about the other side. It's still the same side, in a separate reality. It makes sense to keep the living and dead separate.

I guess so. I knocked on the door, and he answered like he was expecting me. I looked behind him into the living room and saw people sitting on the couch laughing.

At you?

I don't know. Probably. Something was funny. He said, "I could kill you if I wanted and bury you in the front yard with the others." I started backing away, but his eyes were smiling like he knew something I didn't know. Maybe it was a warning. I didn't sleep well last night. I have laundry and cleaning to do.

It can wait.

I hate waiting.

You want everything done yesterday, yet you wait for love like a schoolgirl admiring her crush on the other side of the playground.

I don't want to talk about love. You always bring everything back to love. I had it once, and that's enough.

You can never get enough. It's like water and air; you need a continuous supply.

I need you to quit badgering me.

I'm encouraging you. Okay, back to the dream. What happened next?

I think that wraps it up.

I don't think so.

You always win! You always get your way. Maybe tomorrow we'll psychoanalyze you. I'm the one sacrificing everything for this book, not knowing if I'm wasting my time. I'm the one having to defend myself to a world that knows I've stepped outside the box. Your part of the book is the best. Everyone is going to love you.

They'll love you too, if you let them. If you push love away; it'll get tired of trying and find another home.

I know who you're talking about. He's engaged to her. It's frustrating.

It's more than frustrating. It's tragic to keep soul mates apart.

I need him more than she does.

She needs him, too.

I doubt it.

Don't compare yourself to her; it'll only cause you grief.

I know. Let's move on.

Tell me about the second dream you had.

The dream takes place in an employee locker room. There's a man getting something out of his locker, and Death is standing next to him.

Maybe you should call him Mr. Green Eyes.

I'm standing behind them watching the dream unfold. The man can't see me because I'm there, but not there. You know how it is in dreams.

It's like that all the time for me.

Mr. Green Eyes is wearing a baseball cap because he's trying to be incognito. The dead don't know how to blend in. The hat is from his last victim; he's wearing it to piss me off. I stand there glaring at him, and shaking my head in disgust.

He looks at me, and he hears my thoughts. He knows what I think of his hat, and he smiles. He looks over at the man and nods as if to say, "That's my next victim." I notice papers on the floor and go to pick them up. He gets flustered because I'm interrupting him. He grabs the papers and says, "Those aren't yours." I read the first page; it was a list of doctors.

The next thing I know, the man is done at his locker and heads out of the room. I'm standing behind the table. I want to yell at him, but there's no point; his fate has been chosen. I won't be able to save him. He won't hear me. Death has the power to take life.

It does.

Why did I have to witness his death? What good did it do?

The people you love the most can be taken from you in the blink of an eye. The dream was a reminder that it's not your time.

I'm feeling stressed out and overwhelmed again.

There's time to get everything done. Listen to your body when you get confused. Will this make me feel better or worse? Am I moving in the direction of my dreams or getting further off track?

Good questions.

You know when you're working versus procrastinating. They're not judging you. You're judging you. And if they are, who cares? They have the right to their own opinion. As I've said before, be as comfortable being as you are doing. Sometimes more gets done when you're being than when you're doing.

I don't see how. Being doesn't get me to the store to buy the stuff I need.

You didn't have the energy, yet you got ready and forced yourself to go.

I wasn't feeling well, which made me mad. I wanted to take advantage of the nice weather.

There will be other nice days. Unplug the alarm, throw away the deadline, rest and recuperate. You have all the time in the world.

It doesn't feel like it.

There are times to push forward and times to pull back.

Is there anything else?

Don't be afraid of the unknown; there are beautiful treasures waiting to be discovered. Love yourself first, and everything will fall into place. If you're given the experience of cancer, use it to become stronger. Not everyone gets shaken to the core and has to rebuild their faith.

CHAPTER SIX

Heart of the Matter

I decided to stay home again. The weather is cold and snowy. Hopefully, I can take a walk soon; I'm getting cabin fever. I'm glad you're here to keep me company. (Julie)

I won't be with you forever. (Sunny)

How come?

Our time together will come to an end.

That will make me sad.

Me too.

Do you get lonely?

I like when you stay home and continue our conversation. You're almost done with this book.

I'm glad. I need to complete one project before starting another.

Be proud of your determination; it will pay off.

It's scary to have a book published. I'm airing my dirty laundry.

You don't learn anything from clean laundry because there aren't any stains. Where did the ketchup come from? Was she eating a cheeseburger?

That's funny.

I made you laugh. My job here is done.

You're on a roll tonight, Sunny.

There are many books being written. Keep going back to your original intention. Once the ego gets involved, your mind wanders to money, contracts, and publicity. Sure, those things are important, but they have to come after the hard work. If you don't leave your heart on these pages, the book won't be alive, and it won't touch anyone.

That's my challenge—to be brave enough to share my story. I need to find the strength and courage.

You already have the strength and courage.

I hope so.

Notice how the answers fall from the sky like a snowflake or raindrop. You don't have to force what's meant to happen.

I want reassurance of the outcome.

Do you think knowing everything would make you happy? It's the mystery that makes life exciting. Life would be pretty dull if you had it all figured out.

I don't like ambiguity and confusion.

You're smart enough for both of us.

If I'm so smart, then why do I keep doing stupid stuff?

Every blessing has its curse. You have to take the good with the bad.

Just when I get something figured out, something else falls apart. Is there anything we can count on?

Love will never let you down; it will lift you higher. Love will tell you the truth, even when you want to hear lies. Love is the one thing people can't hide.

How can I let go of my shame? I rinse my hands until they're cracked and bleeding.

You didn't do anything wrong. It wasn't your fault. Stop punishing yourself.

Would you like to hear about my dream?

Part VI: My Spiritual Journey // 151

Sure.

I'm walking up a grassy hill. The weather is pleasant. The next thing I know, I'm pouring the contents of my water bottle down the hill. I don't think I did it on purpose because that was my drinking water. Now, I have to get more water from the store. On my way down the hill, I find my purse hidden behind a rock. When I woke up, I thought about my sun sign, Aquarius, is depicted as the Water Bearer. Maybe the dream was telling me to share my insights.

Allow your creativity to flow, and you'll have abundance.

Could it be that easy?

Yes.

I have a sincere desire to help others.

You've already helped many people. Sometimes, you should've been helping yourself. Before you got sick, it was easier for you to focus on others. Now, you have to focus on yourself.

I'm still not very good at taking care of myself.

Odd you put yourself last.

I definitely need to be first.

You need to receive as much as you give, otherwise you'll be depleted.

I make the simple things complicated.

You do.

What if I'm a terrible writer and I'm fooling myself?

We're not going there again, are we?

I might as well run my fears by you.

Did you hear what you just said? Run your fears by me. Don't run with your fears unless you're planning to leave them in the dust. Your fears make you doubt and then you drop into depression. Do you think you're a terrible writer?

I have my strengths and weaknesses.

Every writer does. Be happy with your style. This isn't about creating the perfect sentence; it's about getting to the heart of the matter. Later on, you can fix your sentences.

I still need to type our dialogue from yesterday. I should've typed it to begin with.

You'll get it typed, don't worry. When you make time, you have time.

⁂

This isn't about me, is it? (Julie)

No, this is bigger than you. (Sunny)

I'm the messenger.

Yes.

How come?

You're ready, willing, and able.

I'm a poor example of what we're teaching.

Because you flush love down the toilet.

That's shitty.

It's one way of looking at it.

Why do I do that?

Because you're scared.

Scared of what?

All that you could have—joy and relief. You're rarely in the moment. You're always looking for an escape. You regret the past, worry away the present, and daydream about the future.

The present moment brings pain.

The present moment is all you have; don't squander it. The moment you chose to focus on the cancer, your whole life changed.

I had to focus on it. Was it not real?

What I was trying to say, the moment you chose to fight the cancer, the way you viewed it, you unconsciously brought yourself a great deal of pain.

How should I have viewed it? I don't think anyone is happy to get a cancer diagnosis. I thought I had a good treatment plan.

You did the best job you could. I'm not saying that, you misunderstand. You could've viewed cancer as something helpless needing love.

Cancer is not a puppy. Now, you sound crazy. Cancer isn't helpless; it wreaked havoc in my body.

You wreaked havoc in your body. You chose sickness. You gave up. What's in the mind gets manifested in the body. Your cells were bombarded with inflammation; the good cells get tired of fighting the bad cells. Eventually, the bad cells win.

Great, so now I gave myself cancer!

More or less.

I didn't want to type tonight, and now I know why.

I'm not pointing fingers.

You're not pointing your ghost finger at me?

I'm trying to get you to see things differently. Cancer becomes strong when you give it strength. There are so many toxins in your environment.

I understand.

Cancer feeds on sugar, stress, and sadness. You have the choice to create miracles or misfortunes. To be a warrior of the light is an awesome responsibility.

I feel like you're pointing your ghost finger at me again.

We're using you as an example because you're willing to be introspective about your struggle. You can't let sleeping dogs lie.

Curiosity killed the cat.

Cancer is taking too many lives. What did your mom tell you today?

She heard about a 23-year-old woman diagnosed with stage IV cancer who will have chemotherapy for a year. She's barely had a chance to live, and now she's facing death. I pray that her spirit stays strong and love protects her from harm.

She will meet her angels like you did.

Do you think I'm ever going to move on with my life?

You'll move on with your life when you've finished the book; it's your duty to the 23-year-old woman.

Do you think she might read this someday? Do you think we can help people?

Yes.

I hope so. Recovery has become my life. Writing is one of the few things that keep me going.

Writing is your current passion.

Writing is my therapy.

Don't be so hard on yourself. People underestimate the repercussions of cancer. You'll focus on the cancer until you stop; it's that simple.

I need to enjoy this moment of creativity; it's better than writer's block.

Part VI: My Spiritual Journey

I remember writing the fiction story; what a great feeling to be consumed with a project. When I finished it, there was definitely a let down because the magic had passed.

Be thankful when the muse is by your side.

I have a question for you. What is anxiety?

Anxiety is pent-up energy. Your worries need some place to go; keeping them bottled up is a bad idea. You've got to work it out, find healthy ways to release stress.

I understand.

Unless you're talking yourself into something, your self-doubt talks you out of it. There isn't much middle ground with you; you're either positive or negative. You rarely take a break or vacation. It takes courage to leave the crowd in order to bring something new back. Your solitude hasn't been for naught.

I hope naught.

Funny.

Are you my spirit guide?

Yes.

I want people to accept you. Angels are seen as a good thing. You first came to me when I was having the bad headaches. Have you always been with me?

More so when you needed me. I've been talking to you for a long time.

I know.

People only hear what they want to hear.

I guess so. I'm living in a brand-new apartment. My fridge is stocked with food. I have safe drinking water. I'm wearing clean clothes. I can't complain too much.

Nor should you; the Universe doesn't like to hear complaints.

Why didn't you prevent my suffering?

I couldn't. I can only show you the way out.

Why does God let bad things happen to good people?

There is no God, not in the sense you mean. He isn't handing out punishments. Look at the good that has come from the bad.

This?

You've changed, even though you like to slip-slide back into your old ways of being. It could've been worse.

I could've gotten pregnant by any one of those guys that I didn't love.

See, you're looking on the bright side.

Yes, cancer treatment was a walk in the park.

At least you still have your sense of humor, and you're trying to make sense of what happened.

I'll never make sense of it. This is just going in circles.

Everything does. No beginning, no end. You mustn't be afraid of success, for it will bring you freedom.

And get people off my back.

Your mom?

She wants me to get a regular job. I want to write and make artwork.

A regular job is not a bad idea; it would give you a routine.

Now, you sound like them.

You need people.

People did this to me.

You did this to you. You asked them.

You're right. I sat there and let them pump me full of poison. I'm trying to forget.

Are you?

Can't you ever give me the benefit of the doubt?

What good would that do? There's no benefit to doubt. Teachers push you to do your best. You'd expect nothing less from me. Are you going to punish yourself forever? Are you going to deny yourself the happiness you deserve?

Yes, I am, until I'm good and tired of this anger and sadness.

Those are not good bedfellows.

No, they aren't.

Too much solitude is not good.

Too much solitude can cause a person to start talking to dead people.

You could be happier.

I am happy.

You're about as happy as the lobsters in the tank at the seafood restaurant.

I'm happier than that.

Not by much. If you don't take care of yourself, the cancer will.

Now, you're trying to scare me.

It'd be hard to scare you at this point, and I don't mean to scare you. I want to motivate you out of this hibernation.

Writers have to hibernate.

And they come out of hibernation when the book is finished.

Well, hello, the book isn't finished! I'm typing it as we speak.

I see that.

I'm never going to finish at the rate we're going. You're wordier than me.

Just make sure you aren't hiding behind your work.

I'm not.

Just checking.

CHAPTER SEVEN

Magic and Miracles

Why is self-love so elusive? (Julie)

The more you love yourself, the more power you have. You're taught to deny what you know and trust what other people tell you. (Sunny)

Why do we have children?

People enjoy the love and warmth a family provides.

No one likes to be alone.

Souls are never done learning. You want to make things right before time slips away, but you make the same mistakes and time slips away anyway.

We keep lying to ourselves until the lies become the truth.

Follow your heart, and the money will come. Do it for the money, and that's all you'll have. It takes a leap of faith. You have to trust the Universe to catch you.

I'm feeling overwhelmed again dealing with the simple things: grocery, laundry, exercise, and cleaning. How can I get everything done? I'm always in a race against time.

You think you're in a race against time. You have all the time in the world. You're setting your schedule. Don't blame the clock.

I have ten things on my to-do list. I feel pressure to get them all done now. I can't decide where to start. I feel like a failure because somebody somewhere probably has all ten things done already. I'm always playing catch up.

Do what's most important first. You'll get everything done, you always do. Who's telling you to get them all done right now? Seems impossible.

My mom. According to her I do everything wrong. I'm too slow.

She's just trying to push you. She wanted you out of the house and on your way.

Out of her way.

Okay, on your way, and out of her way. Your recovery took a long time. She wanted you to speed up so you could rejoin the world. Then she realized you had to slow down because your body couldn't speed up. Then she had to make peace with your passion for writing which isn't a steady paycheck.

Add that to the list of, "Things I did wrong." I'm grateful she pushed me to get better, but sometimes she pushed too hard.

That's when you pushed back and threw your temper tantrums.

I'm 35 going on 13.

Sometimes you are.

I couldn't sleep last night, I hate that.

You had a lot on your mind.

Did you want to talk to me?

I'm always here if you need me, but I will not bother you when you need sleep. Cut yourself some slack; you're further than you think. Your books are in a good place.

I'm not in a good place.

You have good days and bad days.

The manuscript still needs a lot of revision.

And so you'll revise it.

That's what I live for: revision and ice cream.

Do what needs to be done today, and then do what needs to be done tomorrow. Don't cause yourself problems along the way.

I'm worried that I'm not going to be able to maintain my independence. What if I lose everything again?

First of all, you're worrying. Does worrying help?

No.

Secondly, you won't lose everything again, and even if you do, it won't matter.

How come?

You aren't attached to the outcome. You aren't attached to things, careers, boyfriends, and promises. In a sense, you've freed and trapped yourself at the same time. It's okay to have those things; you should have those things. You've pushed everything away so you can't lose them again. You've drained the color from your world. It's the risk that makes it all worthwhile.

So, I should take up skydiving or rock climbing?

If that's what you want to do.

I need to finish this book.

You need a stiff drink.

You're right.

Give yourself a break. You do more than some healthy people do, and they don't beat themselves up for taking a day off.

Lucky them.

Not really.

I don't want to move back in with mom. There's so much animosity between us. She went through the war with me.

She has caregiver fatigue. She has gone above and beyond the call of duty to nurse you back to health.

So, it's my fault?

No, you're good at being sick, and you didn't let anyone else help. You needed to call in some fresh troops, put in the second string. You depend on her for everything. You'll both benefit from time apart. You're doing so much better now.

Thanks.

Choose wellness instead of sickness.

Sunny, you don't have a body. You don't have to worry about breathing, eating, cleaning, exercising, and finding someone to love.

I used to have a body; I can empathize. You'll find him soon enough.

Awesome!

Our conversation is new to you, which is why it feels special.

We're looking for magic and miracles.

We're attempting to go beyond the ego mind.

Which is why it comes out right the first time, and I don't have to pull my hair out in frustration trying to phrase the sentence correctly.

It's why your pen races across the paper trying to capture our dialogue, and your fingers glide over the keys forming the words we've shared.

I enjoy our dialogue, yet I miss real conversation.

Perhaps you isolated yourself because you knew this would happen. You've known for a long time. You could've invited friends over, read a book, or talked on the phone. You don't have to be sitting here typing this.

I know that.

Your isolation, what purpose does it serve? What are you so afraid to hear?

The truth.

Your truth or their truth?

Both.

And what is the truth?

I'm a pathetic loser who waits until her last chance is gone. I push good people away. I ruin my chances. I go back and forth between worshipping and hating him. He's going to marry her, and that's how it's meant to be. He's just my cheerleader. Maybe there's someone else for me.

There is someone else. In time, you'll meet him. When it's time, I should say.

Don't hold your breath. When he marries her, he'll be lost to me forever.

He'll always be your friend.

And I'll always be a good person.

Don't get smart with me. There's nothing wrong with being a good person. I was complimenting you.

That's like telling the person who sat the bench it wasn't a fun game anyway.

You never sat the bench. You can't have it all. You can't be it all, even though you try. Be grateful for the talents you do have, cultivate those, Ladybug. You're the whole package.

Damn right.

No, you're struggling to regain your self-confidence. You doubt your divinity, sweat the small stuff, and sabotage your success. You're one of fate's chosen victims.

You're guiding me now.

Previously misguided, now centered in truth.

I like that.

You'll be free when you choose to be free. You'll stop struggling when you make peace with the past. Even if everyone laughs at you, stand tall and proud, laugh back. Believe things can be different. Learn from your mistakes. Have compassion for those who are suffering.

Does everyone have a spirit guide?

Yes, everyone has a spirit guide. Many people get derailed.

Am I derailed?

Your life changed abruptly, and you didn't get back on track. Oftentimes, derailment is the best thing that ever happens to a person.

I'm not afraid to die. I don't want to suffer. I will miss my family and friends.

Look at death as a new beginning. You'll be here for all of eternity. Do not blame your soul for making you sick to teach you health. Learn what you were meant to learn and then move on.

Why do you call yourself Sunny?

I am the opposite of cloudy. I am the light in the darkness.

Why is the darkness so scary?

The darkness is not so scary. If you really think about it, Julie, the light is more frightening to most people.

How come?

Light makes you accountable for your actions. Light reveals the truth—blemishes are seen, irritations are felt, and feelings have to be worked out.

That makes sense.

People take the path of least resistance. Exercise is difficult so they turn into a couch potato. Cooking is difficult so they eat fast food. Loving is difficult so they turn away. Imagination is frowned upon so they choose science. Feelings are difficult so they become apathetic. Nature is unruly so they use chemicals. Freedom is difficult so people choose slavery. Life is difficult so people choose death.

I'm worried the cancer is back.

Stop thinking about cancer, whatever you think about you bring about. The Universe hears you loud and clear, even if the message gets garbled. You'll end up manifesting the very condition you're trying to avoid.

Alright.

Think about the life you want to have. Forget about the darkness. Cancer is the trash in your mind, garbage in your bowels, trauma in your psyche, and regrets in your heart. Cancer can do a lot of things when it's given fuel. The only thing cancer can't do is love. And that is the power you have over cancer, the ability to love.

On that note, I wish you good night.

Good night, Julie.

CHAPTER EIGHT

Queen of Gratitude

Answering your soul calling is the path to freedom. (Sunny)

It's a big responsibility. (Julie)

Having responsibilities is a good thing.

Do you want to be separate from the cancer book?

No. These topics fit well with your cancer story.

The manuscript is becoming long and repetitive.

Trust that the seeds we've planted will grow and bloom. Even if you get disheartened and face numerous rejections, I want you to keep trying.

I've never been good at finishing things. Why is that?

Fear of the spotlight that you secretly crave. You're hesitant to ask for feedback.

I ask for feedback.

Have you let anyone read this manuscript?

No.

People would encourage you.

I guess so.

You're trying to do it all by yourself. That's crazy talk.

Where is my smart boyfriend when I need him? There've been so many times I've needed to talk with him. He would know what to do. He could help me with this. I'm sure he hates me and thinks I've lost my mind.

He thinks you're bright. He's sad you got cancer.

I bet he still remembers my favorite songs.

You're learning how to stand on your own two feet.

What fun is that?

Believe in yourself. In time, you'll be able to distinguish great from mediocre work.

When am I going to stop struggling? Is this book ever going to end?

Yes, it will end—the book, the suffering. The day will kiss the night. Your head will hit the pillow, and you'll tell the stars good night.

Good. I'm tired of being alone. I want to meet someone and fall in love again. This solitude is for the birds. I hate the wintertime; it's so cold and dreary.

You complain about the heat of the summer, too.

I'm the queen of complaining.

Try to be the queen of gratitude, that might feel better.

I'm ready to trust someone again.

I think it's time.

I thought you were gone. I didn't feel you around, oh, that doesn't sound right. I mean, I didn't sense your presence today.

You usually write at night.

You've been pretty vocal during breakfast. I'm still trying to type what I scribbled in my notebook.

It'll get done.

I hope so.

Choose enlightenment.

Whatever, I'm fine.

You're not fine.

Okay, I'm not fine. My family doesn't understand me. They think I've taken a long walk off a short cliff.

They don't believe in their own potential.

Should I give this up?

What does your heart tell you to do?

Keep going.

Then keep going.

Even at the risk of being a complete failure.

Without risk comes little reward. It takes courage to create something new. Your light is your strength. Can you see in the darkness?

No.

Some families don't provide enough encouragement.

They wanted the best for me. I was the one who was hell bent on ruining everything. They were trying to steer me in the right direction. I could've played soccer in college and majored in physical therapy; it was the obvious career choice. They were right, but I was stubborn. I thought I knew it all. I didn't have a clue.

You didn't want to be locked into a career path until you were completely sure. It had to be your choice and you wanted to feel passionate about it.

Choosing a college major is a big decision. The first two years of college were stressful for me. I lacked self-confidence. I had so much anger inside of me.

I sense an epiphany.

My threshold for happiness is pretty low. I mess everything up so that I can't experience success. I get to be the victim and nurse my wounds. I enjoy my depression. Isn't that the funniest thing you've ever heard?

No. It's quite common.

I deny myself the things I need. I thought I was getting better at this, maybe I haven't learned anything.

Two steps forward, one step back. Catch yourself before you ruin things. You always have a choice. I think you want to change, but you're scared.

I'm a big scaredy cat.

You don't have to be.

I still catch myself not taking the important things seriously.

It takes practice.

There was a part of me that wanted to major in English Literature, but I didn't think I was smart enough. Writing is difficult for me. I worried that I would've struggled through my classes. I could've learned grammar rules and writing techniques.

You would've become a better writer.

Now, I have to teach myself.

At least you're not bound by the rules.

Guess not, since I don't know what they are.

You're funny.

I know.

What issues were you working on back then? (Sunny)

I wasn't working on anything; I was running away. I ran as far as Santa Fe, New Mexico. I ran my boyfriend out of my life. I ran until my dad got sick and then I came home. I realized what a stupid fool I'd been, not that I'm much wiser today. (Julie)

You're wiser today. You've stopped running.

That's because I can't run anymore. My heart is fragile.

Your heart is stronger than you realize.

I just wish things could've been different.

He knew his drinking bothered you.

Why didn't we make him stop drinking? Maybe our silent permission bothered him. Why didn't we force him into treatment? We just stood there enabling him. We had our little interventions, but nothing changed. We didn't care enough.

You cared enough.

We were sending him the message that we didn't care.

It wasn't your job to fix him.

Yes, it was.

No, it wasn't.

Whatever. We should help the people we love, not let them drown.

Sometimes people drown regardless.

That's a depressing outlook.

Just being honest.

Part VI: My Spiritual Journey // 171

I must've looked like an idiot working with recovering alcoholics while my dad was back home in Ohio.

You were trying to understand addiction.

I was.

He wondered why you were so far away.

I've always been a runner.

You were hurting.

I need to stop trying to fix broken people.

I think you have.

I have.

He didn't choose the bottle over you. He lost his ability to choose a long time ago. He had unfulfilled dreams. That's not an excuse, and it doesn't condone his behavior. He didn't want to let you down. He wanted you to look up to him.

I did. I still do. I look for him everywhere.

This is tearing you up again.

Like turning on a faucet, let the crying begin.

At least you're laughing through the tears; that's a good sign.

I don't need anymore signs. We're having another thunderstorm. Thanks for keeping me company.

You're welcome. It's going to be okay.

I don't know how. I feel like I'm drowning again.

It'll get better. This is just a phase. You're so hard on yourself.

I was being mean to myself today. I wanted to cut my arms. I took the trash over and walked for twenty minutes, but I didn't wear a warm enough coat. My mom wanted to get together because we haven't seen each other in awhile. I told her I needed to work on this, and then I felt guilty.

She wants to help you, spend time together, and make sure you're okay.

We both know I'm far from okay.

You have good days and bad days.

Some days, I'm hanging on by a thread. Other days, I'm full of hope. There's a light at the end of the tunnel. I've caught glimpses.

I'm your light for now.

Am I ever going to be in love again?

Yes, if you make the effort and your intentions are sincere. Be careful, your old patterns will resurface. Did the drama-filled relationships get you anywhere?

No, I've learned from my mistakes.

Good.

I have to want to live again rather than ramble on about it.

We're not rambling.

Don't flatter yourself. We're rambling.

We're rambling in the name of recovery.

We're sorting out the mess in my mind.

Do you know why?

The mess in my mind will manifest as sickness in my body.

Exactly. Just don't give up. Please keep trying. Think happy thoughts.

I did a load of laundry this week, so all hope is not lost.

Good job!

Thanks.

You used to be happy.

I used to be a lot of things. I used to be a normal person.

You're still a normal person.

Doesn't feel like it.

Then feel again.

You're so inspirational. How can you be positive all the time?

The alternative isn't an option for me.

How come?

I'm always at a high-energetic frequency.

Must be nice.

Become aware of when you're holding tension, when something doesn't feel right, when you're hungry, when you need to rest. If you go back to being oblivious, not taking care of yourself, your body will let you know.

What's going to happen? You can see my future. I want to know!

You can't know your future anymore than you can change your past. You had to leave everything behind. You feel guilty for no reason. This is your healing. This is work right now and then you'll have to move on.

I'm writing another book; it's a love story. Can I ask you something?

Sure.

Did you have cancer?

I had lung cancer like your father. I was a smoker, too.

Did you die from it?

Yes, I did.

Which is why you're qualified to be my spirit guide, you've been through similar experiences?

I can empathize with what you're going through, and it helps me to help you, if that makes sense.

I think so. You're an angel; it's your job to be helpful.

I also experience healing, even though I'm generally healed.

Did you go through cancer treatment?

I had many rounds of chemotherapy. I fought until the end. I know the hell you've been through. I'm scared that you want to go back there.

Back where?

Back to being sick. You don't have to be sick to be cared for. You can be free.

I'll never be free. I'll always worry about the cancer coming back. Every new ache or pain makes me nervous. I haven't learned anything. I'm stressed out and losing weight. I can't be attached to life anymore; it's too painful.

You're being pessimistic.

I drink soda instead of green juice. Do I really want to live?

Juicing takes effort, opening a can of soda doesn't. You're being lazy.

Thanks.

Remember your cells can only do what they're told. Once they get out of control, it's hard to restore balance, but it can be done.

I feel like I'm wasting away.

I'm here for you.

I'm glad you're here; otherwise, I'd be all alone. This book feels like a baby that's long overdue; it's killing me.

Stay focused. You're almost done.

Amen.

CHAPTER NINE

Moving Forward

What if they only want to hear what you have to say? (Julie)

This is a team effort. Without you there wouldn't be me. (Sunny)

Why am I doing this? Who cares about my cancer journey? What if they're right?

It's helping you, that's what matters. In time, this will help others. Your self-doubt is asking those questions. Strong Julie isn't afraid.

Strong Julie is cool.

How are you feeling now?

Like everything I do is wrong.

How does that feel?

Not good.

Everything you've done has prepared you to be here with me.

What if I'd taken another path?

You did, and you still found your way back.

I guess so.

Even the notebook you bought at Office Depot with your mom and all the notebooks you've bought over the years. You were compelled to buy them?

I like to buy notebooks. I want to be ready when inspiration strikes.

You knew someday you'd write something spiritual, a conversation like this. Even when you were focused on other things, a part of you prepared. The possibility of your gift scared you. You had to wait for the right environment. You knew how serious this would become and the choices you'd have to make.

I was worried people wouldn't understand. Sometimes, I don't understand.

You've had to go against the grain, which creates criticism. You're not wasting your time; time is all you have. And you must return to life.

I don't want to. I want to work on this.

Your life is out of balance.

I'm always trying to catch up to the good opinion of others.

Work at pleasing yourself and then you'll please others.

I'm always a day late and a dollar short.

You're ahead of the times and wealthier than you know. Sometimes, you're even a step ahead of me, and I have to jog to catch up.

Ha! Thanks for your kindness.

Kindness moves mountains.

Today is Saturday. Before cancer, I wouldn't have been home on a Saturday night. It used to bother me being home, but now I don't mind so much. I wonder what people are doing out there on the town?

What does it prove to be out on the town?

Not much.

It only proves you're not home. You could be having a worse time out there.

I choose not to have a television right now so I can concentrate on writing. I miss it sometimes. There are movies and shows I'd like to watch.

You've forgotten how to rest. You're either working or worrying.

That's about right.

Watching television would be more fun than your counting and checking rituals.

I agree.

I doubt you'd turn into a couch potato.

I might. I've been feeling tired when I take my walks. It's beginning to worry me. Maybe I'm just out of shape. I feel like something's working on me again.

You'll have energy when you make energy. Death will leave you alone when you choose life.

I'm tired of hearing you say that. I think Death is going to do whatever he damn well pleases with me. I've made myself sick again. I cried when I was doing yoga because I don't see the way out of this. You won't let me go crazy, will you?

I won't let you go crazy.

How do I start feeling safe again?

Say your affirmations, breathe, and relax. Picture your safe place. When you're consumed with passion, your worries vanish. Have you noticed this?

I have.

You get through the gritty details of the present by imagining a future with him.

A future that will never come.

He deserves a box of chocolates for being your hero. He led you down the path of positive thinking. He's given you so much. What have you given back?

Not enough, I guess.

He's just a man susceptible to the same vulnerabilities. Putting him on a pedestal doesn't give him much room to move. When you love someone, you let him grow and change. You want what is best for him even if it takes him away. You cannot learn everything you need to learn from one person. You need many mentors and mirrors.

Do I come across as needy and sarcastic?

It's okay to have needs. You're meant to protect yourself.

Thanks for being here.

I'm the only person you didn't push away.

And you're not even a person.

That makes me safe.

You can't hurt me.

You won't shatter into a million pieces if you let someone touch you. You aren't as fragile as you think. You need to let your best be good enough. Who cares anyway? People aren't holding up scorecards.

Seems like it. Everyone is peering in the windows judging me.

You're judging yourself, and that's what the world reflects.

I guess so.

We've talked about this. You'll feel strong when you do things that give you strength. Small accomplishments give you confidence.

What if I'm past the point of rescue?

Not possible because you always have a choice.

What if I make the wrong choice?

You won't.

I hope not.

When are you going to stop punishing yourself?

I don't know.

What did you do that was so wrong that you think you need to be punished?

Everything. Existing. Not saving my dad. Cheating on my boyfriend. Doing whatever I want to do. Not being the daughter my mom wants me to be. Falling apart. Taking too long to recover. Getting cancer in the first place. Being as slow as a turtle.

None of that requires punishment. Let yourself off the hook. Set yourself free. Forgive yourself, not because you did something wrong, because you think you have. Forgive yourself for demanding perfection. You're too smart to be struggling like this.

I agree with you.

We're teaching what you need to learn.

What do you need to learn, Sunny?

How to let you go.

I don't want you to let me go.

The book is near completion. You have to return to your real life.

This is my real life.

This is a stepping stone to greater joy. I'm just your spirit guide.

Just. You have just saved my life.

You have saved your own life. I was just a passerby.

I didn't want to type your answer, "How to let you go."

I'm sorry.

Why couldn't you have said, "A hot fudge sundae?"

That's not what I need, Julie. I need for you to get well.

What if I don't?

If you don't get well, you'll get sicker. Those are your two options.

You make it sound easy.

It is easy.

I'm doing a terrible job of taking care of myself. I'm losing weight again. Winter is rough. I'm not getting out enough, and if you leave me then I'll be alone again.

If I leave you then you'll be forced to meet a flesh and blood person and have a flesh and blood conversation. Wouldn't that be great?

Oh yes, wonderful, looking forward to it.

Are you ready to put all that cancer stuff behind you?

It's funny how you bring up stuff from other parts of the book.

I've got my finger on the pulse.

You've got your ghost finger on the pulse.

Just trying to help.

I need to move onto the next chapter of my life.

Your tears create rainbows; it's a beautiful sight.

You must have some sore eyes.

You're one of my favorites.

What if he loves me as much as I love him?

He does.

Does he get scared to be vulnerable?

Yes. He wants to be perfect in your eyes, too. You both want to be respected by your peers and make the world a better place. Like you, he over-thinks everything and doubts his magnificence. He chases his own finish line.

I'm going to reach the finish line if it's the last thing I do.

I bet you will.

Don't believe me?

It's not for me to believe or disbelieve. You talked yourself out of a life that could've been yours.

Don't remind me.

☙

I have a new mantra for you. I think you're ready. (Sunny)

Okay. (Julie)

Well, you're scared to death of living, so we've got to do something. You've created a new prison you can't escape from. Here goes: "The chemo saved my life. I did the right thing. I'm ready to move forward, unafraid of everything I'm trying to control in a misguided attempt to keep from getting sick." And what's actually happening?

I'm getting sicker.

That isn't how recovery works.

I can't even do recovery right.

Maybe you're trying too hard.

And maybe you're just in my mind?

I am in your mind.

You know what I mean.

What does it matter?

I want to know whether you're real or not.

Believe in the sight unseen.

I can see you. I have an idea of what you look like. Do you sleep?

I have no need for sleep, although I do rest sometimes.

I like to sleep in my warm, comfy bed. Anything else you want to add?

You have the ability to create masterpieces, everyone does. It takes a tremendous amount of discipline and devotion. Focus on giving, not getting. Keep fighting.

I'm tired of fighting. Nobody fights this hard.

Do the best you can with what you have.

That's what I do.

Good.

We can always start a new book after we finish this one.

I would like that. I enjoy our time together.

I do, too.

I'm not to replace real people.

It seems as though you know when I'm ready to write.

I can tell when you've made space for me or when you need cheering up.

Sometimes you go on talking when I'm ready to be finished for the day.

You can delay your bedtime when we're on a roll.

Our conversations are special.

Then why do you run from it?

I run from it because it's difficult to explore the topics we're discussing.

It takes courage to heal old wounds.

I agree.

Be happy with your work and seek not adulation. If you write from the heart because you have to write, getting the words onto the page is the reward. Any praise or validation is icing on the cake. Maintain an internal barometer of success. Don't listen to the critics. Create a book that helps people, rather than a flashy book of no substance.

Okay.

There are many people who can relate to your story.

They've been to hell and back?

Yes.

I hope I do hell justice.

Not everyone has what you have. Not everyone can do what you do. Doesn't that make you happy?

Oh yes, it makes me happy that I'm different and life is harder.

Being unique is a good thing. You make life hard.

Something shifted. I can't quite put my finger on it.

You got clear and focused. You left their nagging voices behind.

Why are some people so cruel?

They're jealous or unhappy.

I don't have all the answers.

Sometimes an apple is just an apple. Being introspective all the time can be exhausting. You need to switch gears and have some fun.

Damn right!

CHAPTER TEN

Happy Dancing

You've left out a few things out. We can't end the book without the whole story. I'm not saying you caused the cancer, but you might've helped it along. (Sunny)

I'll never know, and you're wishy-washy. (Julie)

Which answer would make you feel better? You were being healthy and got cancer, or you weren't being healthy and got cancer? It wouldn't matter, you'd blame yourself either way.

I could've gotten cancer no matter what I was doing. I could've been married with kids living in New York painting abstract paintings. I could've been playing professional soccer. I could've been lying on the beach drinking rum.

But you weren't. It's important to understand what causes disease, but at the end of the day you have to let it go and move on.

Alright.

What were you doing before you got cancer?

I was burning the candle at both ends; a lot of people do that and don't get cancer.

A lot of them do. What else happened in the years leading up to it? It takes five to seven years for a single cancer cell to form a palpable tumor.

I was living in Santa Fe going to graduate school. My boyfriend and I broke up. He moved back home to Ohio. I remember the love we had; it still strengthens me.

That's love for you.

Even though we continued to talk, I treated him like a stranger. I regret how things ended. I turned on him. I turned on myself. He was right about everything; he always was. He knew me better than I knew myself. I didn't like the person I was becoming. Losing my support system was the beginning of the end.

You pushed love away.

After we broke up, I was on my own for the first time. That's when I started smoking cigarettes. I know this is horrible to say, but I enjoyed smoking cigarettes; they relieved my anxiety. I dated men I didn't care about, and they didn't care about me. When I had the chance to be with a great guy, I messed that up. I said some really dumb things. I had everything in the palm of my hand, and I threw it all away.

You didn't have to.

I was a silly girl.

What else?

I took the anti-depressant, Zoloft, for several years because I was struggling. Graduate school was more than I had bargained for. I had a full-time course load. I was working part-time at a drug and alcohol treatment center. For my internship, I completed my hours at five different places—from a juvenile detention center to a nursing home. I had zero time for studying or socializing. I barely had time to breathe.

Breathing is important.

That's probably the busiest I've ever been.

Staying busy keeps you out of trouble.

On top of everything else, I found myself a new boyfriend, but he was trouble. How I made time for him, I don't know. When I did exercise, I felt tired and blamed it on the elevation or cigarettes. I was losing weight again. I've always been thin, but this was too thin.

You'll always be thin. You eat healthy, and you're active.

Things were going from bad to worse. I didn't have a job lined up after graduation. I didn't like working at the treatment centers. The only thing I enjoyed was making art and listening to music.

And then what?

I graduated in November of 2006 from Southwestern College with a master's degree in art therapy. My family flew out to visit and attend my graduation ceremony. It was the last time we were all together, before my dad got sick.

This is hard for you to write about.

What gave it away?

The tears welling up in your eyes.

I can't believe how much grief I still have.

Grief is grief no matter how you slice it. The years lessen the sting, but the pain will always be there because you loved him so much. I think we've reached some clarity.

I'm about done seeking clarity. I'm being ridiculous rehashing this stuff. I need to drink an ice-cold beer and forget about it.

That's an option.

I hate this book; it keeps me up until two in the morning and then I look like an undertaker the next day.

We're almost done.

Good.

Maybe that's why you had to write about it one last time: to get it out of your system, to be completely repulsed by it, to stop picking it back up. We've gotten to the heart of the matter many times. You can't put something behind you that you're still processing. Perhaps, you feel ready to move forward?

188 \\ Are You Ready To Put All That Cancer Stuff Behind You?

I do. The weather has gotten warmer. The flowers are blooming. Summer is around the corner. The pool is calling my name. I'm going to buy a new bikini, read some beach books, relax, and enjoy myself. I'm not going to think about recovery. I'm going to be worry free. Well, we all know that's impossible. I'm going to worry less.

That's a great idea! Reward yourself for a job well done. Even though you'll never give yourself credit for what you've accomplished.

I'm going to try. Sunny?

Yes?

Why does it take a whole book for the truth to come out in the final pages?

The truth has been revealed many times throughout the book.

I've had some rough years. I've been through a lot.

You have. We have one more thing to cover.

What?

What were you doing the year before you were diagnosed?

I was working at an insurance company.

And that made sense to you?

At the time it made sense. I couldn't find an art therapy job. My friend, Christen, helped me get the job. I was grateful for her help. I needed to get back out there. It was a great company. I enjoyed my time there, but it wasn't art therapy, and Santa Fe became a distant memory. I left the world of magic for the mundane. I wasn't creatively stimulated.

Why would you be? Insurance deals with facts and figures.

I hung pictures of nature in my cubicle so I wouldn't go insane. In the evenings, I'd make artwork in my bedroom. I did well at the job because I'm organized.

Part VI: My Spiritual Journey // 189

The company was lucky to have you.

I was lucky to have them.

You need to rest; we're almost done.

I love you, Sunny. You're a good friend.

I love you, too, Julie. You've learned well.

What did I learn this time?

You said the three most powerful words in the universe.

I love you?

Yes. The power behind those words is the secret to health and happiness. Say them, feel them, and understand them. Find someone to love who can love you back. That's why you're here, that's what will save you.

I was afraid you were going to say that.

Live for love, and love will live for you.

∽

I didn't realize how difficult it would be to tell my story. (Julie)

It's going to be okay. (Sunny)

I've sacrificed too much. I'm trying to do the impossible.

That's when the magic happens. It's difficult until it becomes simple. A story will come together if you use the right ingredients and allow it to simmer.

We're creating a healing remedy—a nourishing soup.

Becoming a better writer takes practice.

What should I do?

Practice.

What would love do?

Love is ready to have an adventure. Love laughs at herself. Love enjoys a good sunset. Love fixes a yummy dinner. Love buys herself new clothes, fixes her hair, and paints her toenails. Love creates openings in her schedule, windows of opportunity.

This is coming from the person who has me writing at all hours of the day.

Sorry.

You should be.

Hey, that's great, a smile to end the day.

Why are we writing a book and who cares?

I think we've gone over this.

Once or twice.

Do you still need reassurance?

Yes.

We're sharing a message of hope and planting seeds of peace. Somebody somewhere will care. That's not for you to decide.

I was thinking…

There's you're problem, thinking too much.

Can I finish?

Sorry.

I was thinking about how I'm a terrible role model. I never see my friends. I microwave frozen meals for dinner because it's easier. I just need to…

Make a disclaimer?

I've already done that. I hate cancer; it took my dad, and it'll probably take me. I don't want to die. I want to live. I want to be in love again.

You can have those things.

I hope so.

This writing has consumed you.

I've practically stopped talking.

Allow yourself the pleasure of good food and company. Learn to be more flexible because people can't cater to your every whim. Roll with the punches and punch back gently. So, your train derailed, you'll get back on track. I have faith in you.

Glad one of us does.

Too much time alone isn't healthy. You need fresh air and sunlight.

I'm going to take a walk tomorrow. I need to stretch my legs.

Good.

What are the wild things, and how do I dance with them?

The wild things are: elegant unicorns, beautiful fairies, talking trees, chirping birds, twinkling stars, and whispering meadows. Anything filled with God's love is ready to serve you. The wild things are living, breathing expressions of love. You dance with them every time you believe in yourself. When you walk your path, the wonders of creation are revealed to you. We couldn't let the mysteries unfold randomly at anytime for anyone. Only the kind-hearted are invited into the kingdom.

What kingdom?

The kingdom of love.

Is there such a place?

Some call it heaven. I call it home. We give ourselves permission to be happy. We do the work and things get done. We have true freedom. This is paradise.

The map is written on your soul. When it's your time, you'll leave your body and join us.

Really?

Someday you'll be an angel, too.

I'm ready now. I hate it here. I'm all alone.

It's not your time.

I wish it were.

Don't wish that.

I can't help it.

You have to find paradise on Earth first.

I can't. I'm tired. I don't know how. I had it before, now it eludes me.

You can. You have the energy. You know how. You're letting it elude you. Remember everything you've learned. Do your happy dance. Choose the path that brings you joy. Listen to your intuition. Enjoy every delicious bite. The time is now.

CHAPTER ELEVEN

Class Is Over

Did you just add another chapter? (Sunny)

Maybe. (Julie)

It's long enough; you're trying to add the kitchen sink.

Sorry this has taken so long.

It hasn't taken that long, and healing takes time.

I've had more than enough time. I fritter the time away.

You've barely rested this whole time.

I went through the entire winter without one cup of hot chocolate.

When are you going to be good to yourself?

That's the lesson I'm still trying to learn.

You keep putting yourself last.

I had to put the book first.

And when the book is done?

I'm going to buy a new pair of shoes. I've been wearing the same pair for three years. I made a pact with myself that I'd wear them until I got the book done. I wanted to scale down and eliminate choices to make things easier.

My wish for you is a future filled with love and happiness.

Thanks. I still feel guilty for doing what I want. I'm being selfish.

You're so far from being selfish it makes me chuckle. You spend your free time writing a book to help people; I don't think that's selfish.

I want to help everyone; it's not possible.

That's why there are angels. The manuscript is done; you have enough.

Hooray!

Hallelujah!

I've missed you.

I've been around.

Not close enough.

Everything's going to be okay.

I hope so.

Having cancer is a terrible thing, but it doesn't entitle you to be a drama queen and have a pity party for the rest of your life.

I know that.

You sure know a lot.

Ugh.

At least you're smiling.

I'm in a good mood today.

Glad to hear it.

I'm always one step away from crazy.

The best people are.

Good to know.

Julie.

What?

Put the crutches away, you don't need them anymore.

I'm still not 100 percent.

No one is 100 percent. You have unrealistic expectations. Be happy now.

Because it could get worse?

I didn't say that. You're making everything difficult.

Are the angels laughing at me?

We're laughing with you.

I'm not laughing.

You could be.

I feel like all I've done is demonize treatment.

It caused you a lot of pain.

I should demonize my unhealthy diet.

There are many cancer-fighting foods you could include in your diet.

I eat some of them.

Not enough. You have to want to live, not be on the fence. Since you like making lists, you could make a list of them.

Alright.

Make nature your pharmacy.

I'll name some of them; I think people know the difference between healthy and unhealthy food.

Just because they know doesn't mean they make the right choice.

Broccoli, cauliflower, kale, blueberries, blackberries, almonds, walnuts, grapes, avocados, mushrooms, salmon, sweet potatoes, oats, brown rice, romaine, spinach, tomatoes, eggs, pinto beans, flax seed, ginger, garlic, green tea, and honey.

Great list.

Thanks!

How do they help fight cancer?

They slow down tumor growth, encourage cancer cells to die, shrink tumors, boost the body's natural protective enzymes, and flush out cancer-causing chemicals. Adopting a plant-based alkaline diet provides us with vitamins, minerals, and oxygen.

It's a win-win situation.

I need to choose foods close to nature because they are nutrient dense.

You have the power to make yourself happy or miserable.

I'm beginning to realize that.

You're trying to cover everything; it's just one book.

I keep thinking of stuff to add. I don't want to leave anything out.

You need to stop and move on.

I'm afraid to move on.

There's nothing to be afraid of. Be more afraid of standing still.

Did you make the smoke detector chirp last night?

No, just a coincidence; dead battery.

I thought you were sounding the alarm; class is over.

Well, it is for now.

Any final thoughts?

The guy you've been pining over this whole time?

Yes?

He's not the one. If he were the one, you'd be together.

I know that.

How will you fly if you keep clipping your wings?

I understand.

Write a new story.

I will.

Don't run back to the same thing that knocked you down. If you don't learn your lesson the first time, you'll get a second chance.

That's what I'm afraid of.

Don't be afraid.

We were having a stretch of cloudy days and it got me thinking, what's the opposite of cloudy? How do we brighten our mood on a cloudy day? How do we stay hopeful during difficult times? That's you, Sunny. There wouldn't be a book without you.

Aw shucks!

Are we done for real this time?

We're done for real this time.

Thank you.

You're welcome.

Epilogue

We've come so far in such a short time. I see now this is my destiny. Getting married, moving there, or taking that job couldn't have happened back then. I'm where I'm supposed to be, even if it doesn't look fantastic or amazing. Or maybe it does? I'm enjoying the journey, treating myself with loving kindness, being a proud survivor, and looking forward to the future.

And this is the Epilogue, so that means the manuscript is finished. Hallelujah! I seek new adventures to test my courage and prove my fears wrong. The Universe rewards me when I make an honest effort. Happiness sneaks up on me when I'm not looking for it. Love opens the door for me when life feels too heavy. My thoughts create my reality. I choose happy, healthy, wow thoughts!

Each day, we're given the opportunity to love more, dance more, and laugh more. The challenge is to silence the ego and listen to spirit. We have the choice to awaken to our true potential, or continue sleepwalking through life. By sharing my story, I'm no longer the victim; I've become victorious. The wild things keep me company, and I am loved. Through weakness, I've learned strength. Through sickness, I've learned health.

I believe I got cancer to learn about compassion and forgiveness. I'm still learning about them. That's the thing about life: we never get caught up, heal completely, become whole, or reach nirvana. At least, I haven't. We do the best we can with what we have, where we are. And it's usually more than enough and better than expected.

We make mistakes and have regrets. We let people down, we let ourselves down. We lose sleep over silly things. We plan, doubt, assume, fume, and yell at the people we love. We speed up when we need to slow down. We slow down when we need to speed up. We learn as we go, stumbling, falling, and getting back up. The love we've known in the past is possible again in the future. Even if we push everyone away, an angel will appear to remind us that we're loved.

Tonight, I saw the pink sunset reflected in a puddle. That's my silver lining—moments of beauty that make me grateful to be alive. This book is good enough just as I am good enough, always have been, and always will be. These are mere words, and it takes action to put them into motion.

God speed, onto the next adventure!

Afterword

Even though I'm a lover of words, writing doesn't come easy for me. Don't over-think it, my mom told me. Too late, I thought, she knows me well. I'm going to be frustrated until it's done, I told her.

My plan to carve out time to write this book wasn't foolproof. I spent most of my time taking walks, doing yoga, laundry, cleaning the apartment, and fixing meals. Some days, I thought crazy was going to win. I had removed almost every distraction (no television, dating, or alcohol) and still found myself procrastinating. I began to wonder if I truly wanted the closure I desperately needed, and if leaving everything behind was such a good idea, especially when the color drained from my world. Maybe Sunny was right; I'm writing this to find my way back.

I'd already spent countless hours alone with nothing to show for it. I had the wrong idea. You don't give to get; you give to give because love is the most valuable currency. Losing the initial publishing contract was a reality check; it was also a blessing in disguise. The manuscript never would've become what it is now, back then. I gained two more years of wisdom and perspective.

I realized two things: I have the opportunity to say something important, and I can take everything I've learned and use it to help people. What an awesome and terrifying responsibility! Around this time, at a Chinese restaurant with my mom, I cracked open my fortune cookie, and the tiny slip of paper read: "You will make many changes before settling down happily." I joked that it was talking about marriage, but we both knew the Universe was encouraging me to continue.

I spent another year working on the manuscript. I figured out what was missing and new chapters began to take shape. When I added the art therapy and writing exercises, my vision for a recovery manual was complete. I found the lump seven years ago. I've had more than enough time to put the pieces of the puzzle together. Holding onto the manuscript any longer is counterproductive. I need to take my own advice and let it go. The wounded warrior walks away from the battle with her head held high.

So, what happened? I sent out the new synopsis letter expecting to get another publishing contract. Instead, I got many rejections. Choosing to see them as redirections, I decided to hire an editor and self-publish. Not five minutes later, I found Morgan Gist MacDonald on Twitter. Morgan is a writing coach and founder of Paper Raven Books, an editing company. Impressed with her strength, optimism, and knowledge, I thought to myself, "She can help me." Hiring Morgan and her team was a great decision.

If you were able to read this book and found it enjoyable, thank my developmental editor, Jennifer Vander Klipp, for straightening out the mess I had created. She understood my vision and helped me push the manuscript one step further. My copyeditor, Michael Kaltenbrunner, for gently fixing my errors while retaining my voice.

Thank you to Ryan Scheife of Mayfly Design for providing formatting and cover design. Impressed with the quality of work on his website, I knew that I was going to hire him before we had even spoken. Ryan was prompt, professional, and did an excellent job.

This book could not have been written without the help of my mom, Mary Ann, who loves me more than I realize and puts up with more than she should. I love you.

Hugs to my affirmation group for being there from the beginning: Will, Elizabeth, Tracy, and Jan. Thank you.

Special thanks to my family, friends, teachers, therapists, doctors, and nurses. I am grateful for your support and encouragement.

November 2015
Julie Knose
Mason, Ohio

Made in the USA
Columbia, SC
12 July 2020